To my Wife

DYSARTHRIC SPEECH
(SPEECH IN CEREBRAL-PALSY)

DYSARTHRIC SPEECH

(*Speech in Cerebral-Palsy*)

by

EMIL FROESCHELS, M.D.

President, International Society for Logopedics and Phoniatrics

President, New York Society for Speech and Voice Therapy, Inc.

Physician in charge of the Speech-Voice Clinic
Beth David Hospital, New York City, New York

Author of

"PSYCHOLOGICAL ELEMENTS IN SPEECH"

"SPEECH THERAPY"

"PHILOSOPHY AND AESTHETICS OF SPEECH"

"PRACTICE OF VOICE AND SPEECH THERAPY"

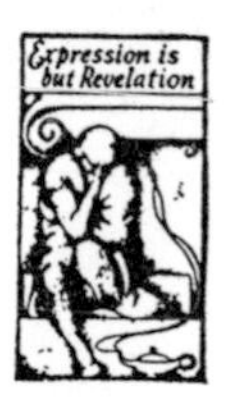

EXPRESSION COMPANY • PUBLISHERS
MAGNOLIA MASSACHUSETTS

PRINTED IN THE UNITED STATES OF AMERICA

FOREWORD

The invitation of Expression Company to write a book on speech improvement for "Spastic Children" and for those handicapped by infantile paralysis was gladly accepted by the writer. To make the book useful to both scientists and laymen interested in this problem meant that some of the more technical discussions of the subject had to be very much simplified. Although this book is devoted chiefly to the symptomatology and therapy of congenital dysarthrias and those acquired in early childhood, both symptomatology and therapy are applicable to dysarthrias resulting from injuries, strokes, inflammations, etc., in adults.

The literature in this field is not very large. About forty years ago the elder *Herman Gutzmann* published a volume called, "Die Dysarthrischen Sprachstoerungen" a part of which deals with those handicapped by "spasticity" due to brain lesions in the motor area. More recently, especially in America, writers have published remarkable contributions to this problem. *T. J. Putnam* has given a most valuable description of the results of spinal cord surgery on athetosis. He has contributed further with *L. Duryea* and *W. Phelps* in the "Symposium on Spastic Paralysis." *Phelps'* interest and practical contributions, especially his orthopedic surgery, are well known to all who take an interest in this field. From another expert orthopedic surgeon, *M. E. Pusitz*, I want to quote some lines which are of great significance for the whole problem: "Messages (from the 'spastics' brain) are still relayed to the muscles, but there is no longer the controlling coordinating action of the higher centers . . . . . . When the message is sent out from the brain, the impulse breaks out with an explosive effect, following not set pathways, but seemingly breaking up into subdivisions at one time." *Pusitz* also describes useful exercises for relaxation. *H. Fagan*, in two publications, outlines not only a practical way of speech development, but mentions also the influence of previous muscle exercises. *S. D. Robbins* has given a thorough description of the various kinds of dysarthria and also stresses the great importance of relaxing exercises preceding the speech training. Also well worth mentioning is a self-description written by a college graduate spastic and the accompanying article by *Palmer* who warns against trusting the results of routine psychometry which may be futile and fallacious if used to determine the potential ability of the particular case. *Dr. Earl Carlson*, a spastic himself, gives valuable advice concerning the psychological treatment of his fellow-sufferers. None of the important American texts on logopedics fail to take into account the problem of helping the dysarthric.*

A word about the question of nomenclature, namely whether the expression, "Spastic Children" should not be changed to "Dysarthric Children." In this book the use of the word dysarthric is imperative as we deal not only with patients whose muscles are overcontracted but also with those whose muscles are too flabby. The suggestion to use the term dysarthria has been made in other publications by the writer and by others.† Another plea is made here to eliminate the word Spastic at least from the field of speech.

---

*_L. E. Travis, S. M. Stinchfield-Hawk, R. West, L. Kennedy_ and _A. Carr, S. T. Orton, L. Raubicheck_ and others.

†_Fentay, Pusitz._

CONTENTS

CONTENTS — *Continued*

First Chapter

SOME RELATIONS OF THE CENTRAL NERVOUS SYSTEM TO VOLUNTARY BODY-MOVEMENTS, ESPECIALLY TO THE SPEECH FUNCTION

The human brain, compared with the brain of animals, differs chiefly in greater development of the cortex. The cortex of the human brain is relatively larger, showing more convolutions and deeper fissures than that of animals. According to authorities the progressive formation of convolutions provides man with new and greater faculties. The formation of fissures appears to be the basis of a close junction of several functions on the one hand, and a separation of functions on the other. Areas separated by fissures are, to a certain degree, independent of each other.

An example of this fact is the so-called anterior central convolution of the brain, which is partly separated from other areas by the fissura Rolandi posteriorly and anteriorly by the anterior central sulcus. The central convolutions are not sharply defined in the brain of hares. In cats and dogs they are separated from the other parts of the brain by shallow fissures. The fissures are deeper in monkeys. In man the separation from the surrounding brain is still more exact and sharper.

Such anatomical characteristics, together with experimental and clinical experience, denote some of the principal differences between man and animals. Movements dictated by will and controlled by reason, are much more indicative of man than of animals. More than three-quarters of a century ago *Fritsch* and *Hitzig* have shown that electric stimulation of different foci (points) in the central anterior convolution of the brain of monkeys produced contraction of different muscles and of muscle-groups respectively, throughout the body. Analogous results were obtained by similar stimulation in the human brain. These experiments eventually resulted in the "localization" of the muscles of the face, mouth, pharynx, larynx, neck and so on down to the toes, in the anterior central convolution. At present we have a kind of guide or map which indicates these localizations. (See Fig. 1.) (See: *C. Sherrington** and: *Penfield* and *Rasmussen*†.)

Place an electric pole in the lower part of the anterior central convolution, allow the current to pass, and you will observe a contraction of the eye-lids.

**C. Sherrington:* Selected Writings. 1939. p. 411 ff.

†*Penfield*, W. and *Rasmussen*, *Th.*: Vocalization and Arrest of Speech. Arch. Neurol. and Psychiatry, 61:21 Jan. 1949.

Stimulate electrically the highest point of this convolution and the toes will contract.

If the central convolution on one side of a human brain is destroyed, for instance by gun shot, permanent paralysis of the voluntary muscles

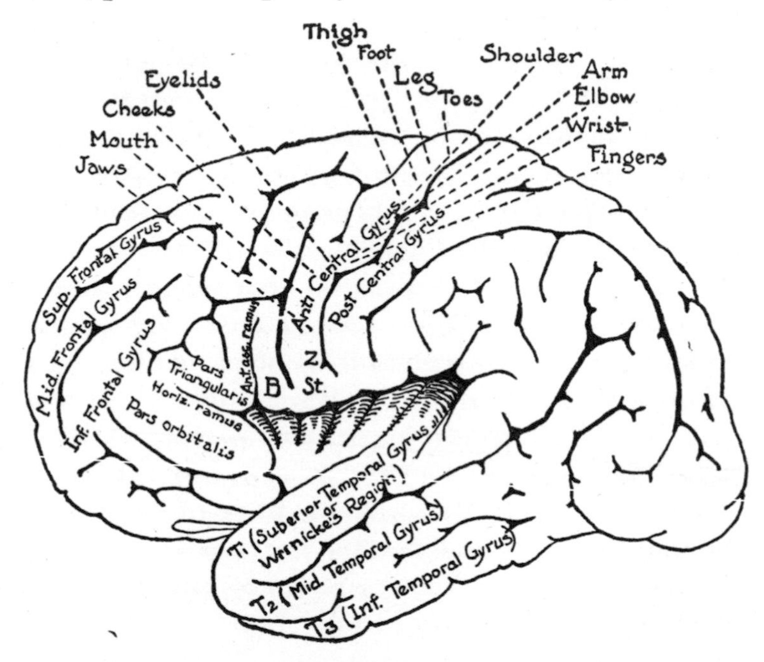

B = Broca's area St = Vocal cords Z = Tongue

Diagram of the Principal Lobes and Fissures of the Human Cerebral Hemisphere Viewed Laterally

Fig. 1

of the opposite side of the body will occur. The same effect may result from a paralytic stroke or a tumor compressing this part. The nerve-fibres connecting the muscles with the central convolutions cross the middle line of the brain and the spinal cord respectively; therefore, paralysis will be manifest on the opposite side of the body. Only the forehead is innervated from both sides, and may therefore remain mobile though the other voluntary muscles of one-half of the body are paralyzed.

An experimental lesion in the anterior central convolution of the brain of a monkey results in a unilateral paralysis only if the monkey is permitted to remain quiescent following the operation. If it is stirred and agitated it will immediately begin to move about in the cage. Extirpation of the anterior central convolution on one side of a dog's brain will not result in paralysis, and the animal will be able to move about and to run, at least after the shock of the operation has disappeared. These facts prove that animals have other powers of movement in the central nervous system not possessed by man. These sources consist of several centers situated in the deeper parts of the brain which are not subject to will. They are still present in man, but are evidently controlled by the higher centers. In other words, the actions of the muscles of the face and limbs, and some muscles of the thorax depend on the will in man. In animals they are at least partly instinctive.

A person who has sustained a lesion of the brain or a stroke is often able to walk again, though the arm and hand remain paralyzed. Walking and moving the hands are certainly voluntary actions in man, but the actions of the hands are more complicated than those of the legs. Many of the functions which the hand performs must be taught, such as writing, sewing, painting, the use of knife, fork and spoon. A baby can walk before it has gained a high degree of control over the actions of its hands.

Language and speech also belong to that category of human actions which depend upon training. One may be sure that a child so isolated that he never hears speech will begin to walk and will learn to use his hands, but will not speak a language.

Observations on brain lesions show that restoration of the function impaired by a lesion of the central nervous system is in relation to the degree of difficulty with which the faculty was first acquired. In addition those parts of the brain which deal with functions acquired by special education seem to be more vulnerable than other areas. In this connection an observation of the famous English neurologist *Jackson** is worthy of mention. He found that cramps during an epileptic seizure began very often in the thumbs and index fingers. These are the fingers used in writing,

*"Selected Writings of Jackson, J. H.", London. Editor: J. Taylor, Hodder & Stoughton, 1932.

drawing, sewing, painting and similar skilled movements.

In his book "Applied Physiology,"† *Wright* refers to electric stimulations of the brain (area 6B). "Electrical stimulation . . . produced rhythmical coordinated movements of the lips, tongue, mandible, larynx and pharynx. Epileptic attacks beginning in this area commence with the same type of movement — chewing, licking, swallowing, grunting." The reader will recall this quotation when he reads the Chapter describing the use of the chewing method for dysarthric speech.**

Summarizing it may be said:

1. The central convolution of the brain in man is characterized by a higher development than that of animals.
2. The portions of the brain which are joined with functions resulting from special training are the most vulnerable.
3. The functions linked with the most vulnerable part of the brain have the least possibility of restoration.

†*Wright, J.:* "Applied Physiology." Oxford University Press, 1935, p. 84.

** See also: *Penfield, W.* and *Rasmussen, Th.:* "The Cerebral Cortex of Man." The Macmillan Company, New York, 1950. p. 217.

SECOND CHAPTER

CONSIDERATIONS OF IMPROVING FUNCTIONS DISTURBED BY BRAIN LESIONS

At first glance the restoration of a function disturbed by brain lesions seems to be beyond hope. The layman may expect that such restoration depends upon the regeneration of nerve cells and nerve fibres. However, the regeneration of the *central* nervous system is excluded if actual destruction takes place. Some forms of stroke and many brain injuries result in a blood extravasate and edema that compress the brain. This may prevent the functioning of the compressed part, in some cases only temporarily. If blood and edema are rapidly absorbed the brain may recover, and the function may be restored completely. Frequently one area of the brain tissue is definitely destroyed and other parts may recover after the re-absorption of the blood extravasate. In some cases no restoration takes place. Fortunately other sources exist which assist the re-education of the function. A *psychological treatment* is frequently very efficient. As a rule, in persons unable to achieve desired results with the usual amount of will or innervation the function completely ceases.

The author had under observation many soldiers suffering from brain injuries who were totally aphasic. Sometimes a psychological treatment changed perfect aphasia into partial aphasia, or even into dysarthric speech. It was evident that such soldiers, who were really aphasic on account of blood compression and edema of the brain, continued to be dumb after the removal of the blood extravasate. The reason for this was *their belief* in a permanent loss of speech.

It is one of the most difficult and most interesting diagnostic tasks to distinguish between psychogenic speech impediments and those conditioned organically. The above-mentioned fact has great significance for the dysarthric child. It is well known that children acquire speech by imitation. If an organic deficiency hinders them in attaining their aim they may pursue one of two ways. They will either remain dumb, or they will endeavor to imitate, but with inadequate results. Sometimes anatomic conditions do not justify or explain the failure to imitate satisfactorily. There are a variety of causes entering into this mal-function. One of them is a psychological deviation. The child, discouraged by his comparatively futile attempts, enjoys building his own speech ("Autonomic Children's Speech," *Eliasberg*).* Another source may be over-use of those muscles or muscle-parts which are easy of movement, and neglect of those muscles which are difficult of movement.

Determination of the cause of mal-function reveals an avenue for therapy. Exact investigation and careful examination of the different muscles participating in the speech act will show the way to special treatment. *Generally speaking, one must first try to strengthen the weak or paralyzed muscles, and if necessary to produce relaxation of others overwhelming in power in order to permit a workable balance.* In Chapters VIII and IX a more comprehensive description of the methods employed for this purpose will be given.

Another possibility of improving the function lies in the fact that the central nervous system contains numerous neurons which may replace those destroyed. The substituting neurons are those which were engaged but little, or not at all, in the formerly normal function. Some examples from other phases of the science of speech correction may serve as illustrations. Normally the visual sense participates only to a limited degree in the acquisition of speech, though a normal baby may observe visually movement of the mouths of people speaking around him. Children especially gifted visually (optic type of *Charcot*) are more interested in visual

---

*III Congress der internationalen Gesellschaft für Logopädie und Phoniatrie. Wien 1929. Publisher: F. Deuticke, Vienna, Leipzig.

observations than other psychological types. Yet the relatively slight influence of the visual sense on speech development becomes evident when we learn that blindness never prevents the spontaneous development of speech. The fundamental investigations of *Dr. Sara Stinchfield-Hawk** demonstrate the influence of blindness and severe loss of visual acuteness on the occurrence of speech impediments. Nevertheless, there is no comparison between the influence of blindness and the destructive effect of congenital deafness on the spontaneous development of speech. It is well known that in dumbness as a consequence of deafness speech may be developed by the "oral method." This method appeals to the visual and tactile senses of the child. Both senses may compensate for hearing to a marked degree. Here we have a substitution of two types of neurons(visual and kinesthetic) for other types (the acoustic neurons), the former physiologically little or not at all concerned with the formation of the damaged functions. Also in many cases of dyslalia (*e.g.* lisping) the optic and the kinesthetic senses help to correct the disorder. Another very interesting and important field which exemplifies substitution of neurons are kindred forms of aphasia. (See Chapter IV.) The visual and kinesthetic methods may also apply successfully in dysarthric (spastic) speech.

---

*Speech Pathology: 2nd Edition, Expression Company, Publishers. Magnolia, Massachusetts.

THIRD CHAPTER

BRIEF SURVEY OF THE PYRAMIDAL AND EXTRAPYRAMIDAL TRACTS PARTICIPATING IN NORMAL SPEECH DEVELOPMENT

In the first chapter of this book we have dealt with the anterior central convolution as one of the most important areas of the brain concerned with speech. From this area many thousands of nerve pathways go down as a part of the so-called corona radiata to the capsula interna. (See Fig. 2, 3.)

The capsula interna is a narrow space between the nucleus caudatus and the thalamus opticus on one hand and the globus pallidus of nucleus lentiformis on the other. It may be mentioned that in the inner capsule the motor nerves of the face are localized on top, while in the central convolution they lie deeper. The fibres after passing the inner capsule cross partly in the medulla and partly deeper in the spinal cord. All these fibres belong to the *pyramidal tract*, and are joined to those peripheral nerves that innervate the voluntary muscles of the face, neck and thorax, the abdomen and the extremities.

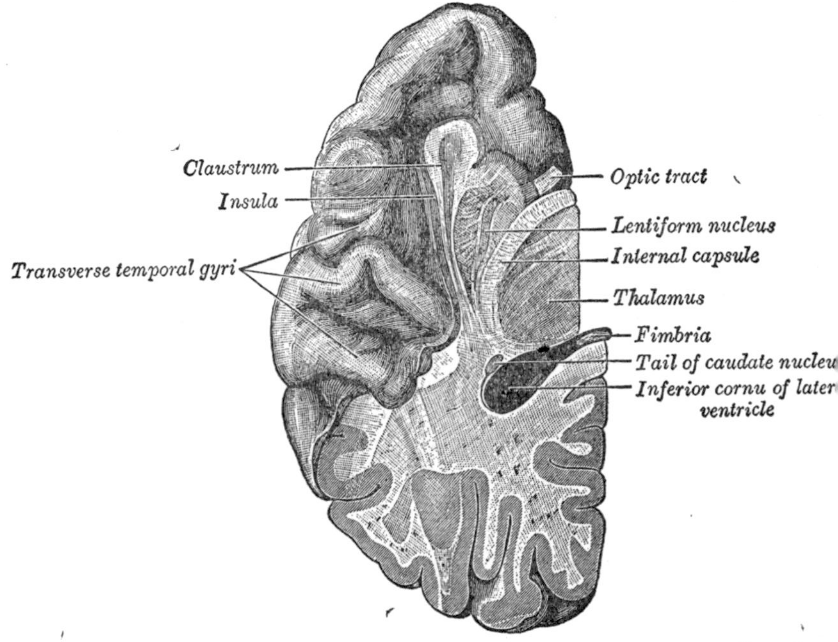

SECTION OF BRAIN SHOWING UPPER SURFACE OF TEMPORAL LOBE. (Gray.)

FIG. 2

Although rigidity certainly may be a sign of a lesion of the pyramidal tract, and thus may be localized there in the spastics *Putnam** says that this opinion is no longer to be maintained so strictly, and *Buchanan*† also suggests that the

---

*Discussion to B. H. Balser "Spastic and Flaccid Hemiplegia of Cerebral Origin." New York Neurol. Soc. and The N. Y. Academy of Medicine, Section of Neurology and Psychiatry. The Archives of Neurology XLVIII, 2. P. 340.

†"Pathology of Chorea," The Journal of Pediatrics. May 1948, pp. 555–557.

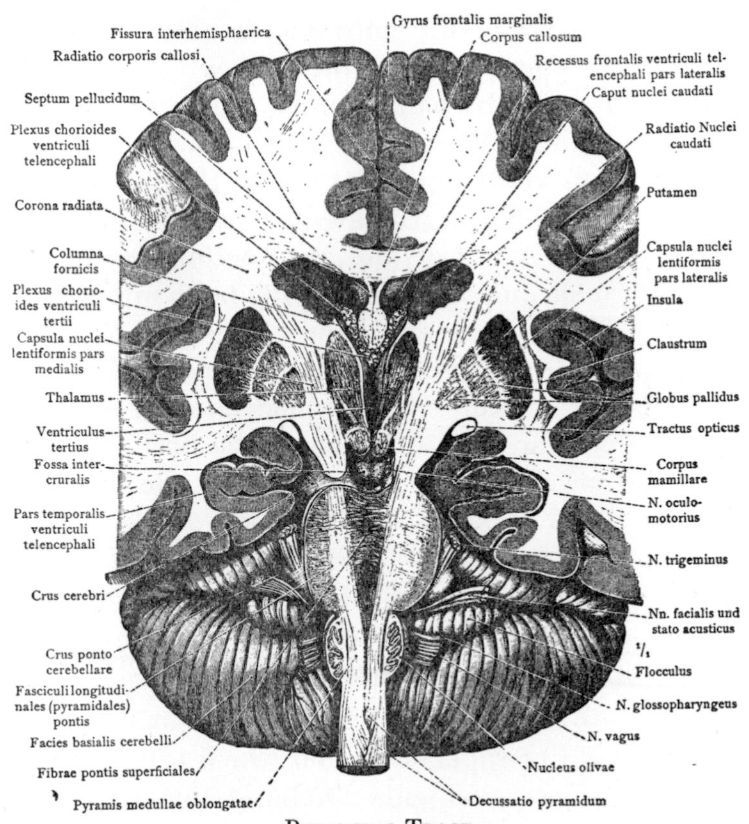

PYRAMIDAL TRACT
(Capsula interna capsula nuclei lentiformis pars medialis)
FIG. 3

central cortex may be the level at which choreatic movements originate. (See: page 41.) These movements have been considered before the consequence of a lesion of the extrapyramidal tract.

Some tracts of nerve fibres originating in centers deeply located in the brain are of the greatest significance for body movements and posture. There are four different pathways. They are called the *extra-pyramidal tracts.* The first runs from the red nucleus below the thalamus into the spinal cord, ventral and lateral to the pyramidal tract. These fibres regulate the permanent contractions of muscles; the contraction normally present in all muscles of the living body are called *tonus.* These fibres also help to regulate the co-ordination of muscles. Two other important pathways lead from the corpora quadrigemina respectively from the bridge (pons) of the brain to the spinal cord. They are responsible for the correlation of visual impulses with the movements of the body. The fourth tract connects the vestibular apparatus of the ear with the spinal cord, the thalamus and cortex. The vestibular apparatus is the chief organ of equilibrium. All four tracts are joined with the cortex of the brain which seems to be a kind of supervisor, and which causes inhibition of the movements produced by the lower centers and pathways. There is also a very important connection between the vestibular spinal tract and the cerebellum.

The *cerebellum* provides collaboration of single muscle-groups, also of those participating in the production of speech. A lesion of the cerebellum may therefore become manifest through lack of co-ordination in the breathing, voice-forming, and articulative muscles. According to *Marburg** the cerebellum also provides adequate strength for the muscular contraction. Hence, deficiency in the function of the cerebellum may become evident by unduly weak or excessively strong contractions. Such a state is accompanied by very slow or very rapid movements. All these abnormalities may influence flowing speech adversely. A similar mechanism produces a voice marked by excessive loudness or faintness. *Seemann*† believes that cerebellar lesions are responsible for delayed speech development. Some French writers maintain that the striatum-pallidum which consists of a part of the nucleus caudatus and a part of the nucleus lentiformis is a center of articulation. *Marburg* sees the most important influence of these centers in the regulation of the tonus of the speech muscles. A disturbance in the function of the centers can produce a tonus that is too strong or too weak. *Wilson*‡ describes the speech of striatum-pallidum cases as blurred and lacking every staccato. Malady of the striatum-pallidum often produces chorea which frequently affects a large part of the body, at times also the speech

---

*Der Einfluss des Kleinhirns und der Stammganglien auf die Sprache. V. Congress der Internationalen Gesellschaft für Logopädie und Phoniatrie. Wien 1932. Publisher: F. Deuticke. Vienna, Leipzig, 1933.

†Dégéneration Lenticule progressive. Revue neurolog. 1912. No. 4.

‡See Chapter V.

muscles. A more comprehensive description of this clinical picture will be given later. *Mingazzini*‡ emphasizes the importance of these centers, not only for articulation but also for the normal origin of speech concepts. With this opinion he realizes the fact previously mentioned that the deeper centers are anatomically and vitally related to the cortex of the brain.

The pyramidal and extra-pyramidal tracts are of motor nature. All voluntary functions of body muscles are inseparably joined with *sensory impressions.* These impressions emanate in part from the surface of the body and the mucous membranes of the mouth and pharyngeal cavity, while another source are the muscles themselves. Such sensations are derived from the tendons of the muscles and the periosteum of the parts of the bones to which the muscles are attached. The sensations pass through the spinal cord, the medulla oblongata, the bridge (pons), the corpora quadrigemina, the thalamus opticus, and finally reach the cortex of the brain, where they are localized in the posterior central convolution, the parietal lobe, and the gyrus angularis. There the functions are:

1. Discrimination of stimuli arising in areas of the body mentioned above which concerns intensity (for instance, the stronger or weaker muscle contractions).

‡L'afasia. Roma 1923.

2. Special relationship; that is, whether or not two moving parts are close together.
3. Differences and similarities and recognition of shape — for instance, the shape of the mouth during the emission of a speech sound.

*K. Goldstein** sees the following common symptoms in all the cases of a lesion anywhere in the central nervous system: The threshold rises and excitation is retarded. It takes the patient longer to react. But if excitation takes place it spreads abnormally and lasts abnormally long. The performance of the organism is influenced to a much greater extent than normally by external factors, and finally the "figure" and "ground" relation is blurred.

The respective roles of the pyramidal and extrapyramidal tracts are still subject to debate. The author believes that the extrapyramidal tract delivers, so to speak, the raw material which is "polished" and ordered by the supervising cortical centers. The final work is done by the pyramidal tract and the joined peripheral nerves. *Garol*† refers to a part of the brain just anterior to the central convolutions from which he could elicit electrically a suppression of motor response to

---

**K. Goldstein:* "Aftereffects of Brain Injuries In War." Grunes & Stratton, New York, 1942.

†*H. W. Garol,* "Suppression of Motor Response in Man." Archives of Neurology and Psychiatry, Vol. 51, 6. June 1944, pp. 525–532.

stimulation of the anterior central convolution. In other words, there seems to be located here a center which may work in such a way that the final motor control executed by the anterior central convolution upon the extrapyramidal motion may still be suppressed or diminished.

The spinal cord in itself does not directly participate in voice production and articulation since the laryngeal and articulative muscles are supplied by brain nerves. But the innervation of the breathing mechanism is, in part, concern of the spinal cord from which the intercostal nerves derive. These nerves supply the intercostal muscles and stimulate their endeavor for contracting and relaxing which causes lifting and lowering of the ribs during respiration. The spinal cord is of motor and sensor nature. The motor parts are chiefly localized in the anterior ("anterior horn") the sensor in the posterior half. (Some motor and some sensor tracts are localized on the sides of the cord.)

The prolongation of the spinal cord, the so-called medulla oblongata, contains the nerve nuclei of six of the brain nerves; four of them, the facial, glossopharyngeal, vagus and hypoglossus nerve are the motor and sensor nerves of the larynx, mouth and pharynx. The facial nerve is the motor nerve of the forehead and the face. The glossopharyngeal nerve supplies the pharynx and the posterior part of the tongue sensorically. The pneumogastric nerve, the motor and sensor nerve of the larynx, is said to participate in the motor supply of the soft palate, and innervates sensorically the lowest part (root) of the tongue. The hypoglossus is the motor nerve of the tongue and the pharynx. Affection of any one of the nuclei is inevitably followed by degeneration of the corresponding nerve. This form of degeneration is characterized by definite symptoms especially related to the electric excitability of the nerve. These "signs of degeneration" do not arise with injury to the pyramidal or extrapyramidal tract of the brain.

The nerve cells in the anterior part of the spinal cord seem to play a nutritive part since their destruction is followed by atrophic states of the corresponding muscles.

Fourth Chapter

THE LOCALIZATION OF SPEECH IDEAS IN THE BRAIN (APHASIA, APRAXIA)

It is well to present here a brief description of the localization and function of the speech centers in the brain, since some spastic children suffer from lesions of these centers (aphasia and/or apraxia). To conserve space, and to avoid repetition the writer refrains from elaborating on this point, and refers the reader to his texts *Psychological Elements in Speech** and *Speech Therapy** for comparison. (A brief survey of aphasia and apraxia follows at the end of this chapter.) Comparison by analogy aids understanding, hence let us compare the centers and pathways previously mentioned with draftsmen and workmen under the supervision of "architects." They are given the ideas, and their task is to perform the work of building a structure, following the plan of an "architect." The nerve centers, called anterior, central convolution, striatum-pallidum, thalamus, opticus, cerebellum and the different pathways, under normal conditions are ready to conform to the plan of the architect, but they are unable to design the building. We shall now introduce the architects to the reader. Fig. 4.

*Expression Company, Publishers, Magnolia, Massachusetts.

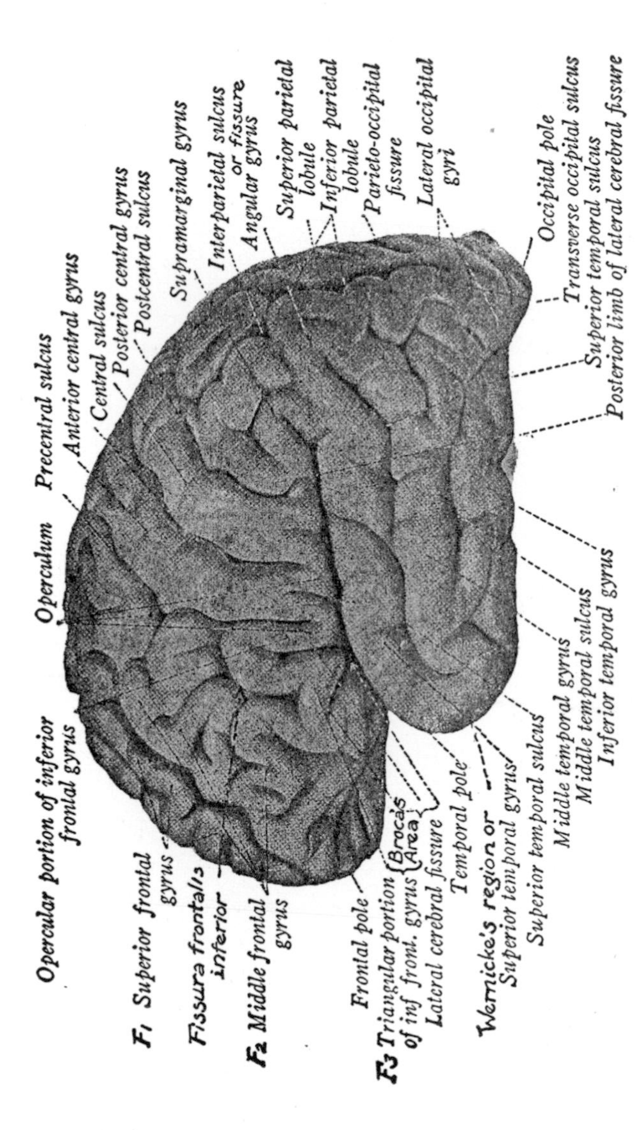

FIG. 4

LATERAL VIEW OF THE HUMAN CEREBRAL HEMISPHERE. (Sobotta-McMurrich.)

In our simile there exists a constructing-firm with a number of architects. One of them is the *acoustic speech center* receiving impressions from the environment. In other words, this center is that part of the brain necessary for the reception of auditory speech — spoken words. This center (*Wernicke's*) is localized in the uppermost convolution of the temporal brain and is stimulated again and again from the moment of birth, since people speak frequently in the environment of the child. *This center has the faculty not only of receiving words but also of recording them in memory.* Later when the child begins to speak he is able to awaken in memory and utilize the remembered words. Another architect in the constructing-firm receives a message that an acoustic image — a recalled word — is to be pronounced. This architect localized at the base of the third frontal convolution (*Broca's* center) has the capacity to develop a plastic plan by which the speech organs can be moved to the positions they must assume to produce the desired words. Both of these architects are actively engaged when one tries to imitate a foreign language which he does not understand. In this instance the speech-hearing center must function to receive the word from the environment and record it. Likewise the second architect must simultaneously devise a plastic plan for the production of the words. When the plan has been deferred to the clerks and workmen in the following order: anterior central convolution; corona radiata; inner capsule; thalamus; striatum-pallidum; cerebellum; lower pyramidal tract; peripheral nerves and the speech organs, the words can finally be produced. Neither of the architects will understand the meaning of the words uttered by the imitator; nor will the child or the person who repeats the words of a foreign language know the meaning of the words pronounced. On the other hand, if a child or an adult learns the meaning of a word some other architects are directing the activity. If a child or an adult sees an object like a chair, a table, etc., without knowing its name they will first recognize its form and perhaps its purpose. The form is perceived through an optic or incidentally a kinesthetic impression. Every optic impression is localized in the *optic centers* located in the occipital brain. *The center for kinesthetic impressions* is located in the posterior central convolution, the parietal brain and angular gyrus. These centers must participate if the architects are to make the word "table" understood. Occasionally the olfactory center collaborates in the understanding. For instance, in recollecting the smell of a rose. Strictly speaking, *to know a thing does not necessarily mean to know its name, and to know a word does not of itself imply knowledge of the thing meant by the word.* The several centers that participate in the knowledge of a thing, with the exception of its name, are called the *transcortical center*. *Only a knowledge of a thing, person or action, etc., associated with knowledge of its name establishes understanding of a language.*

Spontaneous speech is distinguished from imitation by the fact that in the former the transcortical center receives the first impulse. From there the stimulation goes to the auditory speech center, then to *Broca's* center, and finally to the "clerks" and "workmen." If a person repeats what another has said the first stimulus will work on *Wernicke's* center. From there two simultaneous stimuli run to the transcortical (for understanding) and to *Broca's* center (for repeating).

Two important features of the central speech mechanism must be mentioned. First, that in right-handed people *Wernicke's* and *Broca's* centers are localized in the left hemisphere of the brain, and in left-handed people in the right hemisphere. Second, that the psychological types of *Charcot* influence the part that the centers play in speech production. If an individual is highly gifted kinesthetically *Broca's* center may stand in the foreground and the acoustic word-pictures may play a secondary role. At times the optic center which receives and retains the visual concepts, for instance, how to move the mouth, may become the most important central factor in speech production (optic type).

It is extremely difficult to determine the psychological type of a small child. In our special field — dysarthria of children — that determination seems to be unimportant, because in every case we have to appeal to the kinesthetic and visual senses. In educating normal children we must be considerate of the psychological type, since the use of the more strongly developed sense will aid them to learn more easily. For instance the visually gifted child will acquire and retain the subject matter far better if he can read it than if it is presented to him orally.

The three "R's" are engaged in part with the speech centers as they are usually taught orally. It is questionable whether silent reading is not performed through the medium of invisible speaking movements. In addition to the speech centers the visual center in the occipital lobe is engaged in reading; in writing the visual center as well as the center for hand movements — anterior central convolution — are involved.

Studies of *aphasia* belong to the most complicated subjects of neurology and psychology. The difficulties rise chiefly from the fact that brain lesions, which are responsible for aphasia are different in every case; hence it presents a manifold clinical picture. There is no less differentiation in psychological types. Thus, the possibilities of variations are indefinite. The speech therapist and diagnostician will face those difficulties only in patients whose speech was fully developed before sustaining the brain lesion. In dysarthrics most of the time we have to deal with cases in which brain lesions are responsible to a degree for *retarded speech development.* Clinical experience has proved that some "spastic children" have speech impediments that are not the result of defective articulation only, but are also due to lack of understanding or to a deficiency in the function of one of the speech centers.

It will not be difficult to understand the types of aphasia that accompany dysarthric speech. If *Wernicke's* center is affected there is a deficiency of understanding in varying degrees from slight to complete absence. As has been shown, a lesion of *Wernicke's* center prevents understanding by rendering the patient incapable of receiving words spoken by another, a defect known as *word-deafness.* (This clinical picture should not be confused with deafness, since word-deaf patients obviously hear, as they react to noise and tones). Another cause of failure to understand is interruption of the pathways between *Wernicke's* center and the transcortical center. Patients of this group are characterized by "*parrot speech.*" They repeat words one says more or less accurately but they do not understand their meaning. That both *Wernicke's* and *Broca's* centers are functioning is indicated by the fact that the patient has the ability to repeat words spoken to him.

All types of aphasia characterized by faulty understanding or its complete absence are called *sensory aphasias*. *Motor aphasia* is the inability to speak despite relatively clear understanding, provided the dumbness is not caused solely by severe peripheral paralysis of the speaking muscles. A lesion of *Broca's* center, or of the pathways connecting *Wernicke's* center with *Broca's* is the anatomical cause. Care must be exercised not to confuse *motor aphasia* with dumbness due only to severe peripheral paralysis of the speaking muscles.* ("Receptive" and "expressive" aphasia are terms frequently used for "motor" and "sensory" asphasia.)

There is another group of disturbances resulting from lesions of the central nervous system a consideration of which is important to the therapist of dysarthric speech. These disturbances called *apraxia* are distinguished by erroneous concepts or total absence of ideas concerning handling of objects though the muscles may be only slightly paralyzed or totally unaffected. For instance, a patient with *apraxia* capable of moving and controlling the arms and hands is unable to employ a tool or utensil of every-day use. If given a comb he may try to write with it, if presented a

*See: Jeanette O. Anderson: *Aphasia and its Treatment in* "Twentieth Century Speech and Voice Correction." Editor E. Froeschels. Philosophical Library, New York, 1948. And: E. Froeschels: "Psychological Elements In Speech." pp. 3–64. Expression Company, Magnolia, Mass.

drinking glass he is at a complete loss as to its purpose and as to what he is to do with it. If we recall our analogy of the guiding idea and the "architect" in speech performance, we can better understand the tremendous influence of a guiding idea on the performance of any action whatever. For instance, our motor-aphasic patients are not speechless due to paralysis of their muscles, but because they fail to receive guiding instructions as to their movements. The apractic patients are unable to utilize correctly objects and things not because their muscles are paralyzed but due to the fact that they do not receive from the "architect" ordering instructions, for the performance of the action. *K. Goldstein*† has given a clear and workable grouping of the several forms of apraxia, classifying them as *motor. ideative, articular-kinesthetic* and *amnestic apraxia.* The motor type comprises the simplest movements, such as pointing, clenching the fist and imitative actions. Amorphous movements also appear, having no definite form. Ideative apraxia destroys the concept of action, and from our discussion it is clear that failure to receive an outline plan or "blue print" of an action to be performed renders impossible purposeful and co-ordinate action by *any* limb. Simple movements are less disturbed than more complex ones, and imitation is unaffected or only slightly affected in contrast to motor

†Ueber Apraxie. Medizinische Klinik, 1911.

apraxia, while amorphous movements are not present. Some present-day writers deny the existence of articular-kinesthetic apraxia. *K. Goldstein* says: "Such patients are able to perform such complex actions as lighting a cigar; at least the succession of partial acts in such complicated movements is intact, but the partial acts themselves are carried out very defectively." Amnestic apraxia is characterized by only temporary loss of capacity for handling and utilizing objects and things. Now the different forms of apraxia certainly originate in defective centers, but the localization of these centers is still debatable. The possibility of the existence of apraxia in a "spastic child" should be remembered constantly if his skill is less developed than is to be expected from the degree of paralysis present.

Treatment of Aphasia and Apraxia

If we keep in mind that aphasic and apractic patients lack the guiding ideas of speech and action respectively, we shall understand that we must provide them with these ideas. A normal child hearing speech changes his acoustic impressions into "plastic speech ideas" (*Broca*) by means of innate skill. If this skill is lacking it is impossible to succeed in teaching the child by the auditory method, that is, by giving instructions through the medium of the ear. To help us we must call into play other senses: the visual and the kinesthetic. A valuable aid is to show and demonstrate the position of the mouth during the production of single sounds. The use of a mirror is often a practical expedient, since by this means the patient is able to compare the position of his own mouth with that of the therapist. In many cases it is necessary to guide and control the lips and tongue with fingers and spatula. (See Chapters IX, X.) In other instances it is essential to give the patient tactile impressions of the air leaving the mouth and nose, by having the patient's hand feel the explosion and friction of the air which accompany the production of different sounds. In nasal sounds the patient can feel the vibrations on the nostrils with his finger-tips.

At the beginning of the treatment no particular sound is to be preferred, since only the individual clinical picture can give the necessary guidance. If, by chance, during effort to establish the production of a given sound another not as yet practiced or drilled upon is uttered, the therapist should at once seize upon and practice through repetition this accidentally produced sound, and thus endeavor to establish its fixation.

Reading and also writing are, as a rule, disturbed in cases of aphasia. Sometimes the specific centers for these two functions are out of order due to the same trouble that has damaged the speech centers. But it may happen that the reading- and the writing-centers are normal and that the aphasic patient nevertheless cannot write or/and read correctly, because when a person learns these skills he is taught to associate every letter, syllable, word, etc., with the corresponding sound or sounds. In other words he thinks of or pronounces the sound when he writes or reads the letter. (This holds also for "silent reading" especially if the pupil belongs to the motor-kinesthetic type.) All that may seem to concern only people who could already read and write before they became aphasic. But it is understandable that damage to the speech centers will also hinder the aquisition of reading and writing skill, chiefly because of the intimate connection between reading and writing on the one hand and speaking on the other (always with respect to the psychological type). To treat alexia (reading difficulties) we use single letters each of them printed on a separate card on which there is a picture of the appropriate mouth position. It is not possible to discuss here thoroughly whether in teaching reading one should begin with letters or words. For alectics one should start with single letters, proceed to syllables, words, etc., especially to such words that are spelled phonetically. That is to say, words pronounced according to the pronunciation of the specific sounds of the letters in that word (*e.g.* "letter" is really the sum of the specific sounds of all the letters l-e-t-t-e-r). Only later should one proceed to the pronunciation of aphonetically spelled words, *e.g.* "culture." This word does not sound like c u l t u r e but like cultshur. Sometimes it is good to offer the single letters in different colors for example a in bl*a*ck, ee in gr*ee*n, i in wh*i*te, etc., thus forming smaller groups. This formation of smaller groups makes it easier for the patient to remember the letters because there is a smaller number from which his memory has to choose. If one prints b l a c k in black, r e d in red, the patient, if he sees *e.g.* k may remember that he saw it printed in black and will therefore have to choose only among five letters to remember what k means, that is how to pronounce it.

In agraphia (writing difficulties) it is advisable to use an analogous system. If one starts with printed letters the paraphernalia will be the same as that described above. If one starts with or proceeds to written letters the cards showing the corresponding mouth position should also show the written form of the letter.* In many cases the therapist will have to guide the patient's hand for a shorter or longer time.

The therapeutic procedures for agraphia and alexia must be modified according to the degree of difficulties in every case. Fundamentally it will be right to use the single letter method in every case of even slight difficulties which are encoun-

---

**K. Goldstein* recommends "tracing on a pane of glass under which the pattern of the letters are placed so that the patient can see and copy them." "Aftereffects of Brain Injuries in War." New York, Grune & Stratton. 1942.

tered frequently in dysarthrics. The psychological understanding of the therapist will have to find the way of training appropriate not only to the single patient but also to his frequently changing conditions. Experience has shown that the same patient is at times in a more "analytic-synthetic" and at other times in a more "Gestalt" mood.† In other words he will be able one day to read and write whole words as unities and on another day only by spelling them.

The problems of writing and reading in dysarthrics will not be taken up again when speech treatment is discussed (Chapter X) so the reader is reminded to refer to this chapter.

In *sensory aphasia* the type of treatment depends upon the clinical form. In "parrot speech" one must endeavor to open the pathway from *Wernicke's* center to the *transcortical center*, and for this we use simple colored pictures of objects, animals and persons. To prevent diversion of mental concentration there should be only one picture shown at a time. The therapist pronounces

---

†From various experiences in different phases of human life the author could draw the conclusion that normally three types exist. Some people understand nature better by dividing it into parts (analytic-synthetic method), others by "grasping" nature as a whole (Gestalt method) and only a few are equally successful in using either of them. But this typing is frequently complicated by the fact that a single individual may learn one subject more easily with the analytic-synthetic and another subject more easily with the Gestalt method. Of course lesions of the Central Nervous System will further complicate this attempt at typing.

the name corresponding to the picture and asks the patient to repeat it. Gradually two or three pictures which the child has learned to name may be exposed on the desk or table. The therapist will call for them and the patient will hand him the one named. Slowly the number of pictures which the child can distinguish is increased, and as the names of new objects are fixed in memory he gradually acquires the meaning of more words. From pictures of single objects we proceed to scenes, explaining and stressing colors, actions, and all relationships including time and space. The therapist should not be discouraged if progress is almost imperceptible even after some months of hard and slow plodding, for experience has shown that in some cases, due to the psychological factors* involved, it is necessary to break through an obstructing "mental stratum," before one realizes commendable achievement, and progress from there on will be rapid. This is due, no doubt, to the cumulative effect of storing acoustic word impressions, word-meanings, discriminating and distinguishing between ideas and objects, things and relationships, and above all, securing the interest, attention and co-operation of the patient.

Where *Wernicke's* center is affected we treat the case by asking the patient to imitate a sound in

*With regard to those facts and to some very important aspects concerning the treatment of aphasics the reader may refer to *K. Goldstein:* "Aftereffects of Brain Injuries in War." New York, Grune & Stratton, 1942.

the production of which he is aided visually by mirrors and by kinesthetic impressions. Then the therapist immediately speaks the identical sound into the ear of the patient with the purpose of associating the speech movement with the auditory impression which the sound makes upon the child. Obviously the auditory impression received by one in whom *Wernicke's* center is deficient differs from that received by a normal person, but experience has proven that in these patients the various sounds produce different auditory images. In other words, there is a differentiation between their auditory impressions; an "e" for instance, if drilled upon as described, will differ from an "o" in auditory image. Neither of these characteristic impressions will be identical with the auditory impressions received by a normal person when he hears these two vowels spoken. In the case of the patient they are sufficiently differentiated from each other so that if they are associated in the patient's mind with the corresponding speech movements for their production *the result will be sufficient for practical life.* Single phonemes, sound after sound, sound blends, syllable after syllable, word after word, all must be drilled upon in the manner described. The work is tedious and arduous, but the reward may be that understandable and fluent speech is finally attained by the patient.

Apraxia is treated in a similar manner, and in addition we teach the patient the use of several tools, utensils and things, exercising his visual sense when necessary with the aid of a mirror, and guiding his hands if he does not succeed in imitating repeated visual impressions.

Fifth Chapter

SURVEY OF ETIOLOGY AND SYMPTOMATOLOGY OF DYSARTHRIAS

There is a varied etiology for the many clinical pictures now designated by the name "cerebral infantile paralysis." Its cause may be an injury or inflammation or degeneration — the latter probably on a hereditary basis — of the brain. Furthermore, this injury or inflammation may have been acquired before birth, during delivery, or after birth. What happened in the womb of the mother cannot be determined with certainty. It is assumed that an injury sustained by the mother may affect the embryo. Malposition of the embryo in the uterus, or a deficiency in the amniotic fluid constitute danger for the child. Only rarely will an infectious disease of the pregnant mother be transmitted to the embryo producing inflammation in the brain which may result in scar formation.

Whether the age of the mother or genetic factors are of any importance in the development of cerebral palsy is questionable.*

---

*See: *Yannet* "The Etiology of Congenital Cerebral Palsy." Journal of Pediatrics. 24. 1944, pp. 38–45. *Perlstein, M. A.* "Etiology of Cerebral Palsy." The Nervous Child. 8, 2, April 1949. pp. 128–151.

The brain of the child is normally protected from injury during delivery. The bones of the skull are mobile, and the head adapts itself by molding to the form of the birth canal, but if the head of the child is unusually large, or the pelvis of the mother is malformed or exceptionally small, if the birth canal is too stiff, or if the labor contractions are exceptionally violent, an injurious compression of the head may result. Such compressions may cause, directly or indirectly, a lesion of the venous vessels in the meninges or in the brain. It is most probable that the injury occurs as follows: By compression of the head a certain part of a vessel is also compressed, and by prolonged stasis the vessel will burst under the influence of the blood pressure. In our first chapter we considered the influence of blood extravasates on brain substance.

Seemann and *Precechtel*† determined that children with history of malposition in the uterus show abnormal vestibular reactions, and thus prove the assumption of blood extravasate in the cerebellum. Birth injuries from use of instruments may also damage the nervous system of the brain. Disturbances in the blood circulation of the mother produced by heart-disease, nephritis or eclamptic cramps may unfavorably influence the blood circulation of the child. Other causes of injury are premature separation or abnormal position of the

†"Gehoer und Sprache" Wiener Medizinische Wochenschrift 1930, No. 35.

placenta, or partial strangulation of the child by the cord or sudden pushing of the head toward the ring of the pelvis and prolonged labors, premature birth and incompatibility between mother's and child's blood.

*Joseph Novak's** article on birth injuries of the brain offers an excellent survey and critical judgment of the question involved. Bleeding between dura mater and skull rarely occurs, while bleeding just below the dura mater is very frequent. The latter is caused in the majority of cases by tears within the duplication of the dura running from the inner surface of the occipital bone to the sella turica in the middle of the base of the skull. This blood may spread along the superior surface of the brain or/and down to the medulla, the cerebellum and the spinal cord. But bleedings either of flea-bite size or striped-shaped also occur within the brain substance itself. The damage may comprehend the white parts of the brain or the ganglia, chiefly the nucleus caudatus, more rarely the thalamus opticus. Scar formation and shrinking of the normal substance as well as the formation of little cavities are the consequences.

Recently *Josephy*† described anatomic- histologic findings on 22 brains of cerebral palsy patients.

**J. Novak.* "Beziehungen Zwischen Nerven System und Genitale." Biologie und Pathologie des Weibes. (Halban-Seitz). Vol. V. Part 4. Urban und Schwarzenberg. Berlin, Vienna. pp. 1369–1528.

†*H. Josephy.* "Brain in Infantile Cerebral Palsy." Illinois Medical Journ. Chicago. Vol. 91. 1947.

Five among them did not show any trace of a destructive or of an inflammatory process. "In all the cases one is dealing with a disturbance of the normal development, which goes back to an early stage of the embryonic life. Whether it is endogenous or exogenous cannot be decided." In other words it looks as though cerebral palsy may be caused by factors of an inflammatory or degenerative nature as mentioned above. Similar observations have been made by *Yagi*.‡

The causes of infantile cerebral palsy after birth are not wholly clear. Injury of the head, inflammation of the meninges or the brain, and similar conditions combined with a general infectious disease do not seem to create great difficulties for the explanation of cerebral palsy. But often symptoms of affection of the brain appear without recognizable cause, *e.g.* tumors or cysts of the brain, aneurysmas, and abnormalities in the blood circulation and spinal fluid circulation and production.* Some physicians assert while others deny that teething in itself may produce infantile cramps. On the other hand, it is certain that a simple stomach upset may be introduced by cramps. Cramps frequently appear in the initial stages of infectious diseases in children. For-

‡*Yagi*. "Birth Injuries in the Newborn." Japanese Journ. of Obstetrics. 130. 12. 1929.

*See: *Fay, J.* "Cerebral Palsy." Am. J. of Psychiatry, 102, Sept. 1950, pp. 180–188.

tunately, in most cases they do not occur again, nor do they leave any serious consequences. Only exceptionally will they re-appear or leave evidence of muscular paralysis. Congenital syphilis also is sometimes responsible for infantile cerebral palsy.

Cerebral spastic paralysis does not present a uniform clinical picture. It possesses only one common symptom — spastic muscular contraction, but the degree of contraction and the hardness of the muscles differ from case to case, and even changes will be detected within certain limits in the same patient. As a rule, the deep reflexes of the spastic muscles are increased,† and the muscles as well as the bones of parts of the body affected are frequently reduced in size (atrophic). One-half of the face may be smaller than the other half.

Choreatic and athetoid movements frequently accompany infantile cerebral paralysis. *Chorea* is characterized by involuntary movements, very frequently present, which interfere with voluntary movements of the muscles affected. In some patients choreatic movements are likewise in different portions of the body, while in others only

---

†If a real spastic muscle is stretched by the examiner or by the muscle's antagonist, the so-called stretch-reflex will show immediately. That is to say, the muscle will become rigid. This reflex does not occur in tense athetoid (choreatic) muscles. (*Phelps, W. M.*: "The Care and Treatment of Cerebral Palsy." J.A.M.A., 1938. 74. Nr. 1. pp. 1–16.) See also: *Fothergrill, P.* and *Harrington, R.*: "The Clinical Significance of the Stretch Reflex in Speech Reeducation for the Spastic." J. of Speech and Hearing Disorders, 1949. Dec. No. 4, pp. 353–355.

the mouth and neck are affected. In exceptional cases there may be evidence of chorea only in one shoulder and arm. If the fingers are affected they are obviously restless due to choreatic movements, and this is especially noticeable if one asks the patient to spread the fingers. In severe cases choreatic movements may be violent, but as a rule the spasm of the involuntary movements is slight and the action radius limited. In every case the choreatic cramps are sufficiently strong to interfere with the exactness of voluntary movements, and this fact is of the greatest significance. It is difficult to describe the characteristics of choreatic movements; however, violent ones give the impression of jerking and pushing, while the milder present a picture similar to an irregular wave running through the muscles.

Sometimes choreatic muscles need a strengthening therapy.* (Different observers have described many types of choreatic movements but the author does not believe this indicates the necessity for using essentially different kinds of treatments.)

Frequently there is affection of the articulative muscles, and it appears that a slight chorea of the tongue is in many cases an accompanying symptom of this condition. Examination of the mouth reveals the tongue in a state of perpetual unrest.

---

*See: *Stuhlmueller* and *Schaltenbrand*. "Myographische Untersuchungen." Deutsche Zeitschrift fuer Nervenheilkunde. Vol. 150, No. 1, 2.

On the other hand, the soft palate is not so frequently affected, but should it be the chorea is marked by a sudden rising or falling of the organ. The laryngoscope at times reveals choreatic movements of the vocal cords and the epiglottis. The respiratory muscles are often the seat of this disturbance. With X-ray certain contractions of the diaphragm may be observed. At the present time there is no clinical picture characterizing chorea of the pharynx. However, frequent difficulty in swallowing experienced by patients justifies the assumption of chorea of the swallowing muscles. The whole choreatic syndrome is sometimes unilateral (*hemichorea*), and frequently one side is more affected than the other. In *athetosis* the movements are said to be slow and fairly regular.†

A symptom frequently present in cerebral palsy is "*glossoplegia*" consisting of a paralysis of the tongue, which lies flat on the floor of the mouth. Similarly the soft palate may be paralyzed, and if the patient is asked to say "ah" the soft palate may not rise sufficiently to touch the posterior wall of the pharynx, or it may be totally incapable of rising. In some cases one half may be moved more readily than the other.

---

†*Putnam* (New York Neuropathological Society, Nov. 11, 1941) states that it is very difficult to know where the choreatic category ends and where the atheotic begins and vice versa, while *Phelps* ("Description and Differentiation of C. P." The Nervous Child 8, 2, April 1949. pp. 107–127) wants both of them to be distinguished from each other.

Investigation of the soft palate has necessitated our taking its *movements* into consideration as its state can be determined only during movement. In reality this implies more than simple observation; it requires a *functional examination.* Visual investigation of the other articulative muscles must also be completed by functional tests. (See next chapter.)

Other symptoms of cerebral palsy are flaccidity, ataxia, and tremor. In flaccidity frequently muscles are used which under normal conditions support only very hard work ("emergency muscles"). Ataxia is characterized by the inability of the patient to direct a movement into an intended direction and to control the extent of the motion.

Neurology and orthopedics have long since recognized that treatment of the spastic presents special difficulties as a result of the *different degrees to which the various muscles are affected.* Some are highly contracted and some to a lesser degree, while others are not paralyzed at all, but are hindered in their work and development by their spasmodic partners. Furthermore, if we consider the influence of choreatic or athetoid muscles when collaborating with normal or spastic muscles an immense variety of pathological possibilities becomes evident. Patients who endeavor to overcome choreatic and athetosic movements by holding muscles taut may become accustomed to the tautness, thus stiffening the muscles. As *Phelps** has explained, the result may be a kind of spasticity, but in the beginning only voluntary overcontractions were present. We learn from this fact that not all muscles which act in a spastic-like manner are indeed spastic. *Phelps* is also convinced that with respect to the increased excitability of some muscles a movement of one of them may bring forth violent contractions in related muscle-groups. On the other hand, some muscles hindered in their efforts by several spastic muscles tend to degenerate into a state of flabbiness.

The differential diagnosis between real spasticity and habitual contractions on the one hand, and paralysis and functional flabbiness on the other, is often difficult, but it must be pursued to a conclusive finding. It is evident that discovery of the genuine characteristics of the muscles is the only reliable guide to effective therapy.

Sensory disturbances complicate the clinical picture as well as the therapeutic procedures. For instance, if a child has a pronounced lack of sensation in his hand it may be that he will not use the hand at all, thus presenting a sham paralysis of a limb where none exists. With such factors in mind it is necessary to point to the numerous possibilities exhibited in the composite picture which

---

**W. M. Phelps:* "Management of Spastic States in Children "Broo - lyn Neurological Society, March 25, 1941.

make imperative careful neurological investigations as a basis for successful treatment.

The disease which as a rule begins in the spinal cord but may spread over the medulla oblongata and the brain and which sometimes affects speech neurons is infantile paralysis (poliomyelitis acuta anterior). This infectious disease is said to be the result of an invasion by an invisible virus. It affects especially the anterior horns of the spinal cord. Edema and inflammatory reaction is the first response of the tissue to this invasion. In some cases the affected area recovers completely, in others the palsies resulting from elimination of the inflamed neurons diminish gradually and the final restriction of motility is relatively slight as compared with the initial state. In a third group of cases severe palsy persists after the signs of acute infection (fever, pains, drowsiness, vomiting, etc.) have disappeared, but frequently motility improves later on (over periods of years) by means of permanent physiotherapeutic treatment and specific exercises. These exercises are based in part on the principle of substitution, because visual observation of the gait, arm movements, etc., proved to be successful. The speech therapist uses this help extensively, as will be shown later. We have previously mentioned the affection of breathing in infantile paralysis. At times this affection interferes solely with the speech and voice act. In such cases visual and especially tactile control of the thoracic respiratory movements is indicated (see Chap. VIII).

If the brain is involved the brain nerves are frequently the first to be affected. Palsies of the muscles moving the eyeballs, supporting the soft palate, the pharyngeal and mouth muscles may result. Sometimes inflammation of widely scattered areas of the brain substance occurs. Such clinical pictures called polioencephalitis resemble other inflammatory diseases or injuries of the brain, f.i. the primary inflammation called encephalitis, the infection of the brain by an inflammation of a neighboring area (f.i. the middle ear), meningitis, etc.

Infantile paralysis, if localized only in the spinal cord, as a rule, does not affect sensibility, since sensibility is not localized in the anterior horn cells. But the nutritive role of these cells makes it understandable that atrophic changes in the muscles and even in the bones take place. If the speech therapist has to deal merely with an affection of the spinal cord he may find flabbiness of the intercostal muscles which causes some speech and voice troubles (see Chapter VI). Brain nerve lesions will produce flabbiness or spasms of the muscles supported by these nerves. Polioencephalitic damage of the brain substance alone will result in clinical pictures which are identical with those rising from other injuries of the brain. (*Bouman* and *Schwartz** have pointed out that if there is a difference between spastic paralysis and spasms after infantile paralysis the difference is due to the fact that in the latter the lesions are very close to the anterior motor route of the spinal cord.) In other words all symptoms such as flabbiness, spasticity, chorea, and athetosis as well as aphasic or dysphasic disturbances may occur. These facts entitle us to handle poliencephalitic dysarthria together with the other forms of cerebral dysarthrias in the following chapters.

The first aim in the treatment of dysarthric speech should be the harmonizing and bringing into the greatest possible balance those muscles which participate in the formation of voice and speech.

**H. D. Bouman* and *R. P. Schwartz*. "The Degree, The Extent, and The Mechanism of Muscle Spasm in Infantile Paralysis." N. Y. State Journal of Medicine. Jan. 15, 1944. Vol. 44. pp. 147–151.

Sixth Chapter

THE SPEECH OF THE DYSARTHRIC CHILD

The speech problems of spastic children present an indefinite number of varieties and types. It is doubtful whether a description of a few examples would be of any value. The sensitive ear of a logopedist can receive no impression of "flowing speech" in their oral communications, which in reality is practically devoid of this desired quality. Yet the auditory impressions received from their speech do not afford a clear indication as to therapeutic procedure. We can understand and appreciate in part the numberless varieties of their speech defects if we keep in mind the great host of muscles that must collaborate in flowing speech, and the varying kinds and degrees of collaboration. The picture is further complicated by the fact that the nature of their speech deficiency may change from one moment to another in each and every case. This becomes intelligible if we consider that in every state of fluent speech different muscles may collaborate, or the same muscles, in varying strength and degree. These are not the only reasons for the chameleonic speech pattern presented by patients suffering from dysarthria.

We must keep in mind the sudden speech interference arising from an instantaneous choreatic or athetoid attack. Yet even these functional disturbances do not exhaust the possibilities. As a rule, the speech muscles of dysarthric patients receive stimuli of differing strength in two consecutive movements, while physiologically the change is not apparent. If a normal person says, for instance, the word "pillow" the soft palate will firmly touch the posterior wall of the pharynx during the emission of the entire word. On the other hand, the soft palate of the dysarthric child may drop suddenly, rise and drop again during the production of a series of oral sounds.

Despite the kaleidoscopic character of dysarthric speech it is necessary to present a general description of the most obvious symptoms: *The voice* is often monotonous and characterized by being too weak or too loud, at times becoming so faint as to be inaudible, and it is usually abnormal in pitch. Almost without exception* the tempo is slow and the rhythm is broken. *Vowels* are less affected than *consonants*, but frequently start with the wrong onset (*e.g.* glottal stop). The abnormal function of the soft palate frequently produces *hyperrhinolalia* which may be due to a temporary or a permanent flabbiness. In addition the violent

*Rare cases of the striatum pallidum type sometimes present increasing speed but diminishing strength of voice and articulation while speaking a series of words.

contraction of the soft palate may suddenly induce *hyporhinolalia.* *Breathing,* as a rule, is abnormal in dysarthric patients. Inhalation during speech is generally insufficient and the air taken in is often wasted. Some results ensue from this malfunction, *e.g.*: interruption of the flow of speech through new inhalation, and the voice aspirated to a high degree. *Aspirated voice* reduces the clearness, color and volume of speech. *Excessive salivation* constitutes another speech interruption which induces the patient to endeavor to swallow. Most of these children have great *difficulty in chewing and swallowing,* and are unable to speak with food in the mouth. If the chewing muscles are affected movement of the jaw will be labored and retarded.† *Jacob* and later *Palmer* called the attention of the therapists to "tension athetosis and spastic paralysis in which the mandibular condyle slips from the glenoid fossa instead of acting as a hinged joint, resulting in a cumbersome, slow, unprecise mode of speech."† A partial or total paralysis of the tongue increases the difficulty, since the tongue must turn the bite of food in order to mix it with saliva and to carry it to the entrance of the pharynx in which the swallowing reflex rises. The patient sometimes drops food, fluid regur-

---

†*Jacob, Alfons:* "Pathogenese der Pseudobulbaer Paralyse." Arch. Psych. XIV. Berlin, 1909.

Palmer, M. "Studies in Clinical Techniques." III. The Journal of Speech and Hearing Disorders. 1948, 13, pp. 44–48.

gitates through the nose, and choking is a frequent feature especially in infants. Stress has here been placed upon the difficulties some dysarthrics encounter in eating since it is believed there is a common source of movements‡ for eating and speaking. Furthermore, progress in the therapeutic treatment of one function is accompanied by favorable progress in another. When we treat dysarthric speech we improve the chewing function and the accompanying tongue movements at the same time. Experience that progress in one of the two functions influences the other favorably in spastic children tends to prove the theory of the common origin of both.

Consideration and Analysis of the Separate Functions Involved in the Speech Mechanism

Breathing

In normal persons inhalation is the result of the raising and widening of the thorax with accompanying depressing of the diaphragm. The thoracic cage is formed by the vertebral column, the scapula, clavicle, sternum, ribs, muscles and diaphragm. The vertebral column, the ribs and the sternum are so articulated that the lifting of some ribs

‡*Weiss, D.* and *Beebe, H.:* "The Chewing Approach in Speech — and in Voice Therapy." Karger, Basel, 1950.

is accompanied by a forward and lateral widening of the chest. In this way the thoracic cage enlarges and expands as do the lungs which follow its movement. Owing to the downward movement of the diaphragm which forms the partition between the chest and the abdomen the intestines are pressed down and forward; the chest enlarges downward also. The anterior abdominal wall consisting chiefly of muscles, is mobile, and so largely escapes the pressure. In other words, the anterior abdominal wall moves forward during inhalation in sitting, standing and walking and moves upward if the person lies on the back. Therefore, enlargement of the thoracic cage is combined with the described movements of the abdominal wall. Normally, exhalation is characterized by contraction and dropping of the thorax, rising of the diaphragm, and backward movements of the anterior abdominal wall. Movements of the latter during respiration are sometimes unfortunately termed "abdominal breathing" instead of *diaphragmatic breathing.* In the opinion of the author the name "abdominal breathing" should be eliminated since the movements of the anterior abdominal wall are only an effect of the respiratory movements.

If a person is silent, expansion of the thoracic cage and the forward movement of the anterior abdominal wall synchronize. The period of time consumed in inhalation and exhalation is practically the same. When a person cries, speaks, or sings, or when a normal baby cries the ratio between inhalation and exhalation changes remarkably. The period of inhalation is short and fast while that of exhalation is long and slow. In addition more air is inhaled as a result of speech activity than when one remains silent. *Gutzmann** describes "physiological incongruity" between thoracic and abdominal movements during speech. The abdominal wall sinks before the thorax. *Schilling*† among other writers, reports a lack of physiological incongruity in some forms of central dysarthria.

Respiratory movements are visually noticeable to some degree. *Tactile determination*, however, is more reliable. The investigator touches the thorax with one hand and the abdominal wall with the other. With this simple method the author has found a lack of diaphragmatic breathing in some cases of dysarthria after encephalitis lethargica. The results were corroborated by

---

**Gutzmann, H.* "Physiologie der Stimme und Sprache." 2. Auflage. Braunschweig, 1928. p. 29.

†"Experimental-phonetische Untersuchungen bei Erkrankungen des Extrapyramidalen Systems." Archiv fuer Psychiatrie und Neurologie. 75, 4–5, 1925.

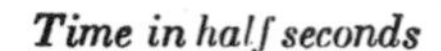

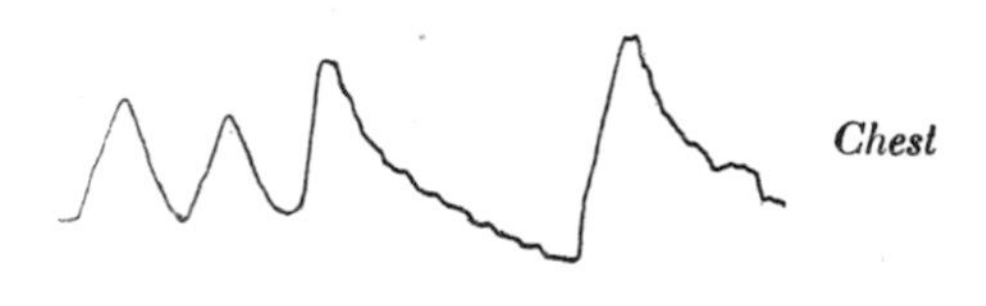

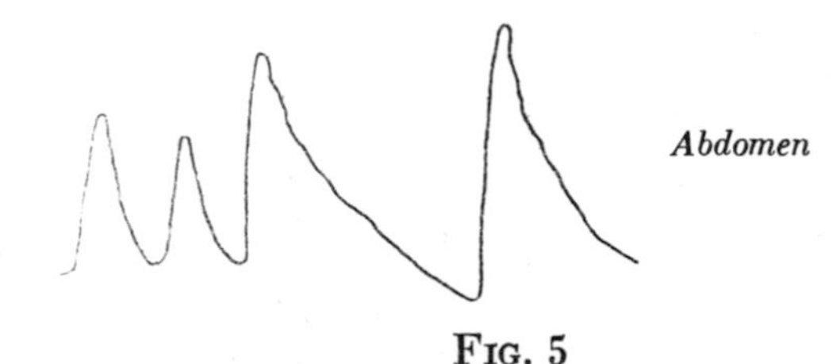

Fig. 5

Schilder.‡ More exact findings are obtained by *pneumography*. Fig. 5 illustrates a normal pneumogram. In silence the ascending and descending parts of the curve are almost equal in length, but when one is speaking the situation undergoes a remarkable change.

The following pneumograms are of dysarthric children and dysarthric adults, the latter having acquired dysarthria through brain injuries. Fig. 6

‡"Zentrale Bewegungsstoerungen mit besonderer Beruecksichtigung der prache." Bericht ueber die Verhandlungen des zweiten Internationalen Kongresses fuer Logopaedie und Phoniatrie. Wien 1926. Verlag Deuticke, Wien und Leipzig, 1927.

Time in half seconds
Larynx
Chest
Abdomen

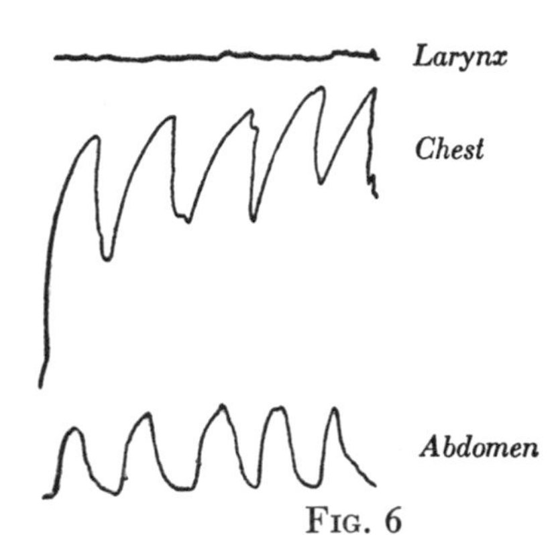

Fig. 6

of a dysarthric man portrays respiration before speaking. The most striking feature is that the thorax does not return to the level of departure; in other words, the patient does not exhale sufficiently. The pneumogram (Fig. 7) was obtained

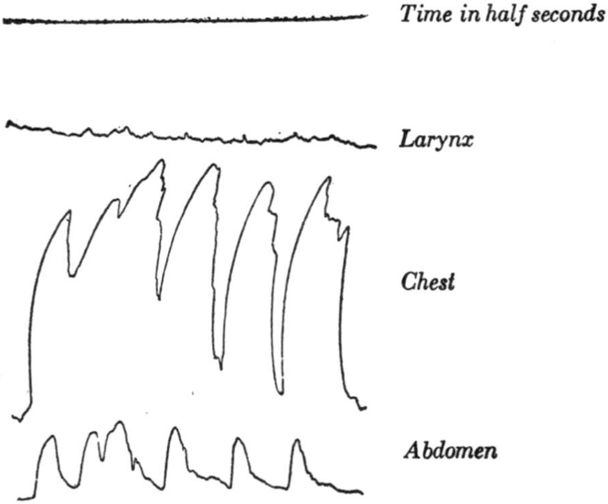

Time in half seconds
Larynx
Chest
Abdomen

Fig. 7

while the patient was speaking. In the first part of the curve the patient inhales before exhaling adequately. The diaphragmatic curve shows the same malfunction. The patient required six inhalations for eighteen words which a normal person speaks with three inhalations. Such pathological breathing becomes most obvious during reading (Fig. 8). The pneumogram (Fig. 9) of another

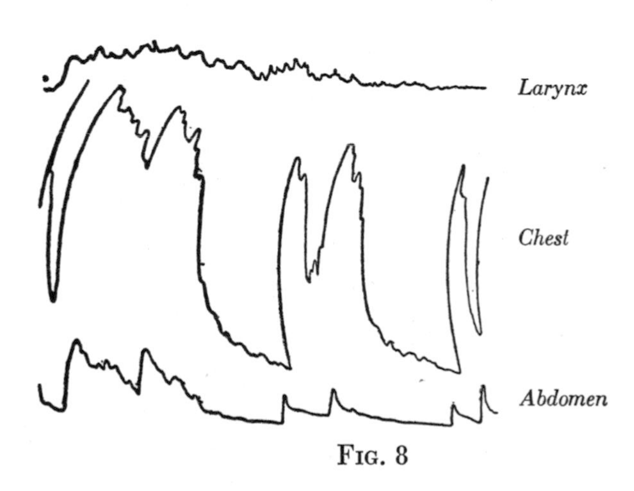

Fig. 8

centrally dysarthric adult is full of different abnormalities. The chest curve begins with deep inhaling, but exhaling takes place rapidly which indicates a waste of air during speaking. The succeeding respirations are very shallow, and do not always indicate normal relationship between inhal-

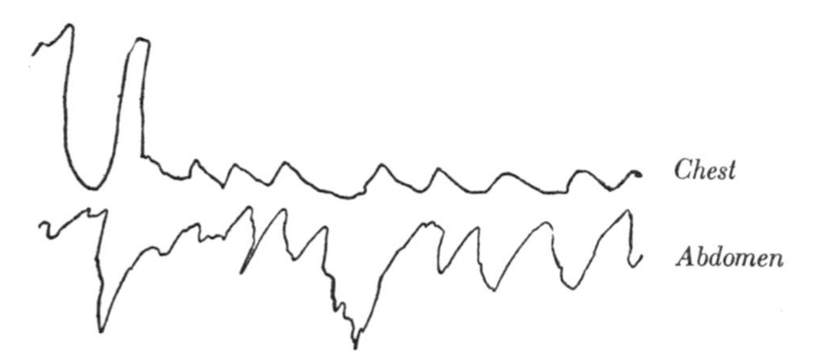

Fig. 9

lation and exhalation. The diaphragmatic curve fails to agree with the thoracic curve on practically every point. Only twice was zero reached in the descending parts of the curve. Most inhalations start after insufficient exhalation. Fig. 10 is the pneumogram of a male patient while reading. Besides numerous other abnormalities the number of inhalations used for only forty-four words is pathological.

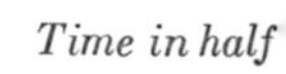

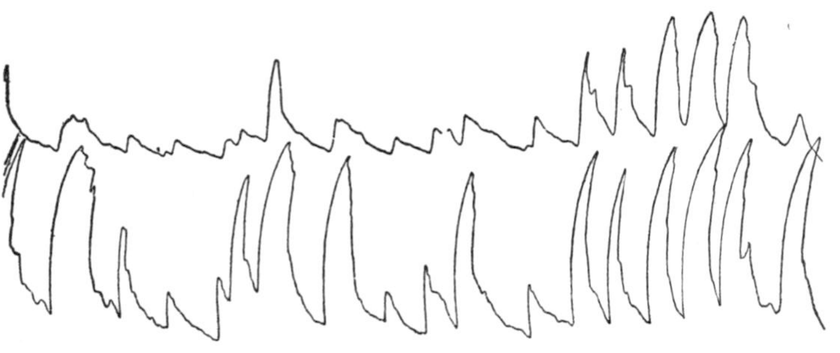

Fig. 10

Summarizing: The most common forms of breathing troubles in central dysarthric patients are the following: Respiration may be affected both during silence and while speaking. Silent breathing is sometimes very shallow, and at other times abnormally deep. Inhalation may occur before the air already taken in is fully consumed. On the other hand, waste of air with accompanying breathy voice is frequently noticeable. There may exist incongruities between the curve of the thoracic wall and that of the abdomen, with the abdominal wall presenting opposite movements to those of the thoracic wall. (*Hull* and *Bryngelson**). In speaking and reading normal incongruity may be absent on occasion or permanently. We may suppose a jittering of the muscles from the numerous peaks contained in the ascending and descending parts of the pneumographic curves. An unfavorable, and even destructive influence of these abnormalities on speech and voice formation is evident. Breathy voice, disturbed modulation, disturbed volume and pitch, may be consequences of pathological breathing. All sounds may be articulated with too much breath, and waste of air will frequently result in insufficient breath for continued speech. This feature is especially harmful to plosive sounds, but also to other consonants, interfering with normal volume. *Hull* and *Bryn-*

gelson saw some patients talk with the thorax constantly expanded.*

The means by which breath (air) may enter the body physiologically are: the nose during silence, and the mouth while speaking. It is not necessary to consider here the influence of nose breathing alone on speech and voice, as recommended by some voice teachers. Even partial obstructions of the nose, as well as dropping of the jaw, may prevent inhalation through the nostrils. It is well known that perpetual mouth-breathing is to some extent harmful. Therefore, our purpose in strengthening the muscles which close the mouth will prove to be generally beneficial. The several categories of disturbed functions which combine and fuse with each other, constitute the basis for the immense variety of symptoms we have previously mentioned. Such impairments will be analyzed when we consider abnormalities in the functioning of the muscles.

Voice

Movements of the larynx are the result of contractions and relaxations of muscles affixed to the larynx and the hyoid bone, and the larynx and the sternum. Fig. 6 shows in the second curve from the top *registered movements of the larynx. The movements of the larynx* are registered with a small

---

**Hull, H. C.* and *Bryngelson, B.* "Speech Monographs." VIII. 1941, pp. 114–121. See: Speech Abstracts 3, 1943, p. 61. C. W. Dow.

metal pan covered with a rubber membrane which touches the Adam's apple and is connected with a registering tambour. Recording the normal movements of the larynx during silence reveals the absence of, or only very feeble but regular movements upward and downward with respiration. These are in part the consequence of elongation of the trachea during inhalation and a shortening of the trachea during exhalation. In Fig. 6 the movements are irregular in time as well as in height. In the next two figures 7, 8, the speaking and reading movements of the larynx also deviate from the norm. Attempts at registering movements of the vocal cords in experimental phonetics have not yet been satisfactory. We must, therefore, be content with a general description of the picture obtained in laryngoscopy. Surprisingly enough, laryngoscopic pictures of individuals with dysarthria do not appear to be pathological as frequently as would be expected when we consider the abnormal voices of such patients. Individuals not accustomed to laryngoscopy move their vocal cords too forcibly. Such excessive innervation is effective even in some cases which normally fail to produce voice at all.

During respiration movements of the vocal cords are often insufficient in dysarthria. To guarantee deep inhalation the glottis which is the space between the vocal cords should be considerably enlarged, but it is most frequently insufficiently opened ~~in dysarthrics~~. The cause for this may be weakness of the openers or a spasm of the closers of the glottis. Normal exhalation sounds like a prolonged H. There is a visible triangular opening of the glottis with a basis of about 2–3 mm. In the case of dysarthrics this opening is sometimes too small, but it is sometimes too large, due to flabbiness of the closers or spasms of the openers respectively.

Since the technique of laryngoscopy influences innervation to a certain degree the resulting picture may not always be characteristic of the regular function of a particular larynx. The author introduced a method which does not change the physiological condition: that is, the auscultation of laryngeal functions. A rubber tube about three-quarters of a cm in diameter is used. To one end a small wooden or metal funnel is adjusted, and the other end is placed in the examiner's ear, who can then listen to the breathing by placing the funnel on either side of the Adam's apple. Normal persons produce a faint, regular sound during inhalation and a harsher one during exhalation. If there is spasticity of the closers or palsy of the openers of the glottis a much harsher inhaling noise is noticeable, the character of which approaches that of normal individuals during exhalation. Such findings during inhalation are indicative of a glottis that is too small, in other words if it sounds sharp as compared with a normal person an abnormally small glottis may be assumed. For auditive comparison of both sides of the larynx the author constructed the "differential stethoscope." Fig. 11. One of the funnels is placed on each side of the Adam's apple. To compare both sides the examiner closes alternately each of the rubber tubes near the funnel with two fingers, which are also used to press the funnels toward the larynx.

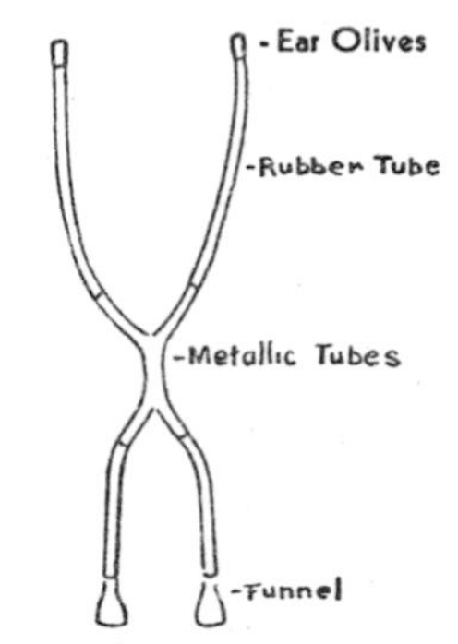

DIFFERENTIAL STETHOSCOPE

FIG. 11

The same instrument aids us to detect flaws in the phonetic use of the vocal cords. In spasticity an initial vowel often begins explosively as a result of a spasmodic closing of the glottis at the beginning of the sound. Such a sudden closure is opened naturally by the exploding air. Physiologists designate it as glottal stop or "*hard intonation*" as compared with a smooth, easy beginning which is called "*soft intonation.*"

As to abnormalities in the voice-production of dysarthrics we must rely chiefly upon our ear. Mention has been made of the pitch which is often abnormal, and of sounds too soft and low or too sharp and high. Inflexion is frequently missing, and often exaggerated, especially in states of excitement. *West, Kennedy & Carr** use the word "tenseness" as most descriptive of the qualities of these voices. Previously attention has been called to deviation from normal volume of the voice. (The author cannot agree with *Rutherford's*† findings that athetoids show more loud voices than spastics.)

To secure a more exact analytical result a systematic examination of the patient's voice is necessary. The first step consists in determining the number of sounds the patient is able to sing. The examiner may use a piano or sing one tone after another and direct the patient to imitate. In excessive degrees of dysarthria the number of tones, which may be called the *compass or range of the voice*, may be severely limited. The higher tones normally depend on a greater tension or stretching of the vocal cords. The pharynx, the mouth, and the nose which are the upper resonating cavities for the tones influence the pitch and

*"The Rehabilitation of Speech," Harper Brothers, New York, London, 1937, p. 109.

†*Rutherford, B. R.*, "A Comparative Study of Loudness, Pitch, Rate, Rhythm and Quality of the Speech of Children Handicapped by Cerebral Palsy." The Journal of Speech Disorders, 9, 3. Sept. 1944, pp. 263–271.

of course the timbre. This has been demonstrated convincingly by *D. Weiss*.* If a wooden or metal tube is placed between the lips and a scale is sung, the voice suddenly breaks at a definite height. Now, if the tubes are of different lengths, and are used one after another, the voice breaks in different pitches according to the length of the tubes. Such a tube is nothing but an immobile mouth. Having this in mind we can understand with *Weiss* that primary tone production may be destroyed or stopped if the tones enter a cavity the form of which is not suited to every tone produced. The mouth and pharyngeal cavity are mobile and instantly adapt themselves to the momentary pitch. In other words, these cavities must change their shape for different tones. If stiffness or flabbiness of the muscles prevent the mouth and pharynx from rapid changes of shape the tone of certain pitches may be distorted or even destroyed. We understand, therefore, that training of all movements of the lips, the tongue, the palate, etc., will not only be favorable to articulation but also to voice production. We may anticipate here by emphasizing the practical values of such methods. It is the chief task of a singing teacher (for normal persons) to increase the voice circumference. All methods and techniques have three common features:

*Zur Frage der Registerbruchstellen. Zeitschrift für Hals-Nasen-und Ohrenkeilkunde. 1932 Bd. 30, pp. 353–358.

1. Training of the muscles stretching the vocal cords.
2. Attempts to influence the muscles indirectly by strengthening and regulating exhalation.
3. Endeavoring to influence indirectly the function of the vocal cords by improving the shape of the upper resonating cavities.

Each of these procedures must be used if we are to correct the voice of the dysarthric child.

The next step in diagnosing voice is to determine whether the patient is able to *maintain a definite pitch for a given time.* It is evident that a lack of this skill may be due to respiratory difficulty or malfunctioning of the muscles of the vocal cords or the muscles in the upper resonating cavities.

Of the greatest significance for normal speech are the so-called "*swelling tones.*" A swelling tone is one in which the loudness may gradually increase or decrease. Individuals with a voice disturbance tend to increase or decrease the pitch while increasing or decreasing loudness, but the normal swelling tone should not be changed in pitch. Swelling tones are frequently used for emphasis in everyday conversation. Involuntary change in pitch will change the meaning and should, therefore, be avoided. Another skill of voice and speech is rapid *changing from one pitch to another.* Children suffering from dysarthria are usually incapable of rapidly changing from one pitch to another. That the spastic child is incapable of regulating sufficiently the loudness of his voice has previously been mentioned. He should be directed also to *sound rhythmically* in different tempi and on different pitches, and for this purpose, the use of a metronome is recommended. What is called *inflexion* or *modulation* of the voice is a combination of the functions mentioned above and will be most unsatisfactory in dysarthric children.

Articulation

Analytical examination of the *articulative muscles* is somewhat easier than that of the respiratory and laryngeal muscles since the articulative muscles are readily observed without the use of special instruments. As a rule, neither X-rays nor pharyngoscopy are necessary for diagnostic examination. This is probably the reason why some neurological symptoms which indicate the condition of these muscles have been detected. We will consider such symptoms later.

The patient's face, at first glance, may reveal trouble in muscular activity, as we have stated previously. For instance, if the jaw is sagging and saliva drooling over the chin, we are instantly aware of malfunction in the muscles responsible for the closure of the mouth and for deglution. Closing the mouth is, in part, the work of those muscles which lift the jaw and, in part, of those which move the lips. Consequently, we must examine both of them in order to localize the site of the defect. Perhaps, the patient can raise and lower the jaw fairly well but cannot close the lips. On the other hand, he may be able to close the lips firmly if the examiner assists him to lift the jaw. Sometimes, spasm of the digastric muscle, fixed to the mastoid and hyoid bone and the lower surface of the jaw prevents the jaw from rising. The same defect, however, may be due to paralysis of the muscles lifting the jaw, masseter and temporal muscles: the masseter fixed to the sygomatic and malar bone and the jaw; the temporal muscle fixed to the temporal bone and the uppermost part of the jaw. The so-called *masseter reflex* is used to indicate some conditions of the masseter. A tongue depressor placed horizontally over the lower teeth is lightly tapped with a reflex hammer

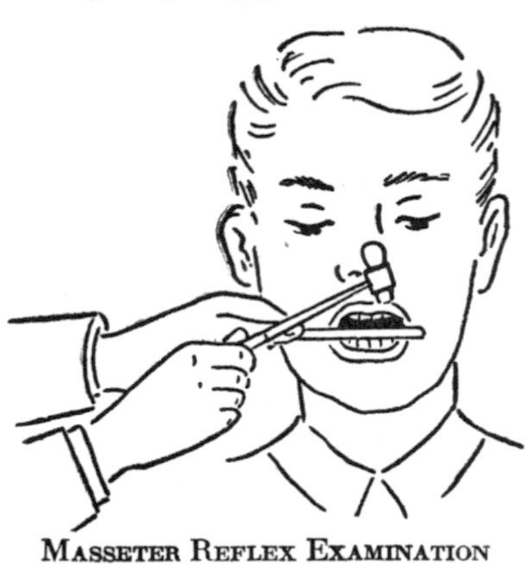

MASSETER REFLEX EXAMINATION
FIG. 12

near both the right and left corners of the mouth. In normal individuals, a short rising of the jaw results followed by a rapid falling. In spastics, however, this reflex is increased and may be clonic. That is to say, several movements follow one tap. At times, the reflex on one side is stronger than on the other indicating that there exists a difference in the excitability of both sides. This difference may be due to a flaccid condition on one side or to spasm on one side or unequal spasms on both sides. If one side reacts normally while the other reacts too feebly or too strongly, unequal reflexes will also occur.

The upward and downward movements of the jaw are especially significant in speech. The examiner should determine the condition of these functions by instructing the patient to elevate and to drop the jaw. If it is impossible for him to do this, a mirror should be used to aid him by visual means. If necessary the jaw should be elevated with the hand in order to ascertain how much energy must be added to the patient's effort, *e.g.*, to find the amount of resistance arising from the digastric muscle. A similar investigation must be made in order to determine the patient's ability to drop the jaw. To obtain information about the state of the muscles which open and close the lips we must examine the capacity of these muscles to draw the corners of the mouth downward, backward and sideward, and narrowing of the mouth as well as protruding of the lips. In all cases of severe disturbance in any of these functions a mirror should be used and the patient assisted manually in order that the examiner may ascertain the extent of the impairment.

The tongue is principally a muscular organ possessing normally a great variety of possible movements. The fingers of the most efficient pianist cannot move as fast as the tongue of a person during conversation. Another property of the tongue is that only the lower part is fixed to bone, while the anterior part of the back, the blade and the tip are free. All other striated muscles of the body are fixed at both ends. This double fixation insures exactness of degree of contraction, and double signals of the momentary position of the muscles to the central nervous system, since tension on both points of fixation is reported. As the anterior part of the tongue is not fixed it is impossible for the central nervous system to get as many messages from this organ. This is the reason the tongue possesses a less accurate sense of position than other muscular organs. The sensation of position is assisted by the sense of touch. For instance, if the tip of the tongue touches the incisors consciousness of the tongue position is keener and more accurate. This factor changes the fundamental diminution of the sensation of place and position.

The examiner can ascertain the state of mobility of the tongue if the patient is asked to protrude it between the teeth, through the lips and out of the mouth cavity, to move the tip gradually to the ridges of the upper and lower incisors, to the right and left corners of the mouth, respectively, to the upper and lower molars, and finally to turn it backward permitting it to press on the soft palate. If deficiency of mobility is apparent the procedure should be similar to that in deficiencies of the muscles of the jaw and lips. A mirror should be used by the patient and the tongue moved toward the desired position by hand or with a spatula. For determining the degree and extent of paralysis of the protruding muscles a piece of gauze is employed to hold the tongue and to draw it slightly forward. In this position it may be examined for flabbiness or spastic resistance of the muscles involved. These muscles are: the geniohyoglossus, the styloglossus, the lingualis, the transversalis and verticalis, and the glosso-palatinus. The speech therapist is referred to recent studies concerning the function of the tongue muscles, by *M. A. Goldstein** and *J. Keaster*.†

The next step in examination concerns the patient's faculty of raising the back of the tongue, and of drawing it backward toward the pharyngeal wall.

---

*"New Concepts of the Function of the Tongue." The Laryngoscope, Feb. 1940.

†Dissertation Presented to Washington University, June, 1940.

If one side of the tongue is paralyzed, or the entire organ is paralyzed with one side more seriously affected than the other, *the tongue will deviate to the weaker side.* This tendency becomes more obvious if the tongue is thrust out of the mouth. Such "pointing of the tongue to the weaker side" results from the counteraction of one side of the geniohyoglossus against the other. The stronger half of the tongue will push the organ toward the weaker side.

All movements of the jaw, the lips and the tongue must be examined with respect to the patient's ability to perform them repeatedly. For instance, the child should be directed to drop and elevate the jaw several times in succession. While the patient is doing this the examiner may make observations; that is, he may find that a movement performed once cannot be repeated, or can only be repeated less accurately upon a second or third attempt. There may be, and most usually is, delay in repetition so that the normal rate may not be reached because of an intervening period. The normal rate for dropping and raising the jaw is about five per second.* Another deviation from the norm relates to the strength of the different movements during iteration. The importance of this point will be considered later. (Chap-

**West, Kennedy and Carr,* "The Rehabilitation of Speech." Harper Brothers, New York, 1937, p. 113 and *Ried, L. D.*, "The Frequency and Distribution of Speech Defects in Spastic Children." Thesis, Syracuse University, 1942.

ter IX.) The examiner will find a metronome very useful in his observations on iterations.

We turn now to the function of the *soft palate.* This organ must also be put through a routine reflex examination. A slight touch of the mucous membrane covering the musculus palatoglossus or of the pharyngeal wall normally provokes retching and raising of the soft palate. This reflex is often exaggerated in nervousness but frequently absent in hysteria. It is also absent or greatly decreased if the sensibility of the area touched is diminished or destroyed. Such deficiencies of sensibility may be caused peripherally but are chiefly due to a central lesion. Another cause of disturbance of this reflex is palsy of the pharyngeal and palatal muscles. If the soft palate does not rise reflexively due to paralysis, it will not move in speech either. On the other hand, it is possible that while this organ functions *defectively in speech*, it may possess adequate reflexive action. To ascertain the speech function of the soft palate, the examiner should look into the open mouth of the patient while he is saying "ah." Normally, the soft palate will rise and touch the pharyngeal wall.

Speech abnormalities of dysarthric cases are as follows:

1. Inability or failure to move the soft palate.
2. Insufficient movement of the soft palate: it may rise but not enough to close the mouth

from the nose. This problem will be considered later. (Chapter VII.)

3. Only half of the soft palate rising adequately; the other half is incapable of movement at all or moves less than the other. In the latter case, the uvula will be drawn toward the stronger side.

*Weiss** found that an active intention not to raise the soft palate may occur (*Active Hyperrhinolalia*). Experience proves that spasticity of the soft palate also produces a similar picture. To make a differential diagnosis between paretic and spastic deficiency in the function of the soft palate, the following test is useful: instruct the patient to utter some vowels in upright position and to repeat them while lying horizontally on the back. *Schlesinger*† describes a diminution of hyperrhinolalia in the supine position since the soft palate sinks down against the pharyngeal wall following the law of gravity. This fact can be used for *differerential diagnosis between paretic and spastic states of the soft palate* as the spastic palate resists the influence of gravity and causes the opening between mouth and nose to persist. *All anatomical,*

**Weiss, D.*: "Eine noch nicht beschriebene Sprachstoerung, Hyperrhinolalia activa." Logopaedie en Phoniatrie (Hague, Holland), 9, 10, October 1937, pp. 87–91. — (*Robbins* and *Robbins* also describe these symptoms in "Correction of Speech Defects of Early Childhood," Expression Company, 1937).

†Wiener Neurologisches Centralblatt, 1906.

neurological and functional investigations must be pursued in order that the examiner may discover the genuine basis of the speech impediments.

Neither the visual nor the auditive control which the examiner may exercise on the movements of the lips and tongue of the patient is sufficiently effective to reveal the causes of the speech abnormalities of these organs. It was necessary to employ an experimental phonetic instrument (pneumograph) in our observations on breathing. To aid in diagnosis, the movements of the larynx were registered during phonation. Therefore, it is essential to utilize graphic methods for minute investigation of the lips and tongue. For this purpose, a very simple and inexpensive device is recommended. A glass tube, affixed to a small rubber ball, such as is used for instillment into the eyes, is adjusted at its other end to a rubber tube. The latter is connected with a recording tambour. The walls of the rubber ball must be thin and easily compressible. The rubber ball is placed between the lips. It may be compressed rhythmically so that the stylus lifts and drops at regular intervals, rising each time to about the same height. In dysarthria of the lips, the examiner will find many irregularities affecting rhythm and strength (height of the elevation). Often with spastic children, the stylus does not move at all. That is to say, the patient's lips have not the strength to compress the rubber ball. Care must be exercised to place the rubber ball between different portions and areas of the lips to determine whether one part or area possesses greater strength than others and hence reveals locations of greater or lesser injury.

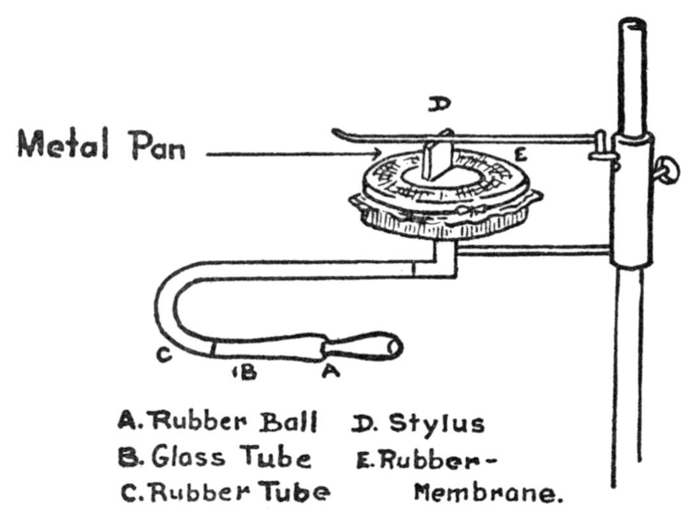

FIG. 13

To register the force and rhythm of the tip of the tongue, the rubber ball is placed behind the upper incisors. This expedient will also reveal a jittering of the muscles, especially if the patient is directed to hold the rubber ball between the lips or between the tip of the tongue and the upper incisors. With the ball held in the mouth of a normal person the curve does not vary after beginning until just before the end of the test. Fig. 14 is a record obtained when the rubber ball was held between the tongue tip and the upper incisors by a postencephalitic dysarthric (a boy 18 years old). The curve consists of many peaks as a result of the trembling and jittering of the muscles

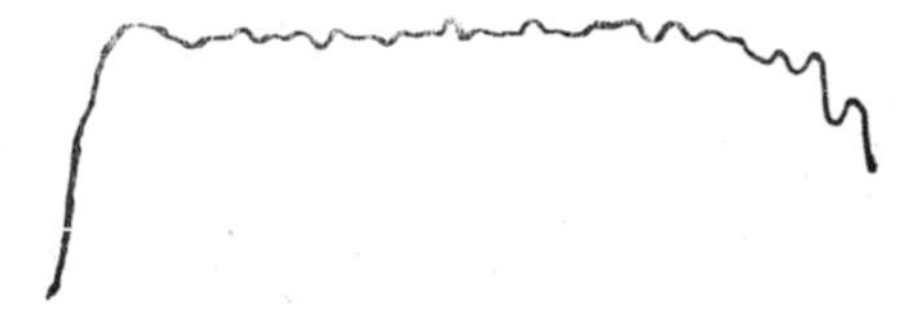

FIG. 14

of the tip of the tongue. It is well to mention here that the same apparatus may be used in therapy. If the patient learns to use his muscles in a more efficient manner he will see progress recorded by stronger and more regular movements of the stylus. This offers not only a means for better control but also stimulates endeavor. For this purpose a kymograph is superfluous, as the patient is able to observe, in the air, movements of the stylus.

If we now proceed to the *examination of speech sounds, syllables and words* we no longer scrutinize separately the motility of articulative muscles or isolated functions of the larynx or isolated respiration. On the contrary, *we determine the coordination of these three functions.* Incidentally, movements of the articulative muscles are the only functions which can be isolated at all, since a definite position of the mouth is inevitable if we are to examine respiration. Furthermore breathing and mouth positions are involved if we are to ascertain the character and function of the voice. Through careful auditive attention, combined with visual observation, the examiner is likely to discover many deviations from the norm. The production of vowels, for instance, may reveal incorrect positions of the lips, tongue and soft palate; inability to maintain a sound for a given time; abrupt interruptions of the voice; pitches which are contrastingly too high or too low; trembling of the voice and excessive movement of the Adam's apple. In some cases the vowels correspond to the vowels asked for by the examiner, while in other instances defective articulative movements will cause the substitution of another vowel sound in the place of one requested. For instance, if the patient is instructed to say A and the jaw and back of the tongue drop Ah will result. U will be replaced by O if the lips cannot be brought sufficiently together.

Pronunciation of B, P and M depends upon a closure of the lips. If the closure is not performed a fricative will replace the sound desired, provided the patient continues his attempt. However, if the closure can be effected it may not be strong enough to produce a plosive sound. Again, B and P will be changed into fricatives. The closure may be strong enough at the beginning but a choreatic movement may interfere and open it prematurely. B is voiced, and therefore, requires for its production a more complicated coordination than P. Sometimes a simpler coordination replaces the more complicated and P instead of B will result. Strangely enough the contrary also happens, with B being sounded when P is intended. This phenomena may be explained by the close relationship between lower air pressure and the vibrations of the vocal cords. Many writers hold that the voiced plosives require less pressure than the voiceless. M may be unfavorably influenced by choreatic contractions or spasms of the soft palate, or by obstructions of the nasal passage.

F and V are normally produced with an articulation between the lower lip and the upper incisors. If the jaw is permitted to drop slightly and the lower lip fails to touch the upper incisors, the resulting larger space between the lip and teeth will not materially interfere with the pronunciation of these sounds. Also, if the lip is drawn up over the upper teeth, the acoustic result will not be greatly distorted. Fricative sounds are generally less vulnerable than plosives. An excessive opening will, of course, make pronunciation impossible. As to the voice the relationship between F and V is the same as that between P and B. Therefore, the pathological variations will be analogous. W may be influenced by the same difficulties in a manner similar to U, and furthermore may be affected by temporary or permanent inability to maintain articulation, exhaling, or voice production, since its pronunciation takes more time than U. WH, a voiceless consonant, is replaced at times by W, and in addition it may be affected by the same distortions as W. The fricative sounds mentioned, at times are emitted like plosive sounds if too strong muscle action takes place.

In the second zone of articulation, D, T and N may be distorted in a similar manner to P, B and M in the first zone. In addition, the tongue may be placed between the teeth. Such position in itself does not prevent plosive sounds, but if the closure is too feeble due to dropping of the jaw a fricative sound similar to voiceless TH will result. If the back of the tongue instead of the tip is raised the sound emitted will depend upon the degree of elevation. If the back touches the palate K, G or NG respectively are produced.

Another fact of general significance may be mentioned at this time. *As a rule all sounds are influenced by the phonemes with which they are connected.* If the patient has in mind a vowel which is to follow D but suddenly substitutes G for D it will take him more time to bring the speech organs into the position necessary for the pronunciation of this specific vowel than it would have taken had he really pronounced D in the beginning, and it is doubtful whether the patient in such instance is successful in the production of the vowel aimed at. The ear is very susceptible to any defective or distorted pronunciation, and the example used here, as the reader will understand, is only one of thousands which might be cited, since every faulty pronunciation may open a vicious circle of almost indefinite circumference.

If the tip of the tongue does not touch the upper incisors, but the blade articulates sufficiently with the palate D, T, and N may not be noticeably changed, but if this closure is incomplete the consonant will resemble a hard or soft S. The defects of S and SH will be considered later.

With L the following faults may occur: the tip of the tongue may be placed between the teeth or pressed too strongly against them; in certain cases the blade may become the articulative part; dropping of the jaw combined with an even incomplete palsy of the tongue may interfere greatly with articulation. In this case, as in many others, a substituting sound may be produced when the correct articulation is impossible. Lateral pronunciation of L, in which air escapes on one side to a greater extent than on the other, is often combined with lateral sigmatism. In such cases L happens to be voiceless, thus resembling the Celtic L that is unilateral and voiceless, but the voice may also fail in L that is not lateral: that is to say, an L which is articulated in the middle portion of the mouth may be voiceless due to a momentary or to a permanent failure of voice in the production of L.

In the speech of those suffering from dysarthria R is often replaced by D, T, voiced S and uvular R. If the motility of the back of the tongue is affected G, K, and NG will be distorted. The plosives may be too feeble as a result of insufficient closure between the back of the tongue and the palate, or the sounds themselves may be replaced by fricatives. Frequently, the glottal stop is used instead of the plosive sounds of the third zone of articulation. This failure is especially harmful to the voice. Intensive closure of the glottis may not only provoke nodes on the cords, but the habit of exerting excessive closures of the glottis is transmitted to the muscles which narrow the pharynx as well as to the articulative muscles. *It is a general experience in the pathology of speech and voice that a malfunction in one portion of the whole apparatus, from the diaphragm to the articulative muscles is, without exception, transmitted to other parts of the speech mechanism.* This will be all the more probable if a central nervous condition stimulates the nerves and muscles to strong spasmodic contractions.

CH, J and soft G are often pronounced as double consonants. For example, observe G in "German" or "ginger", and the G sound represented by DI in "soldier". CH consists of T and SH; J and soft G consist of D and voiced SH. Now if one or both of the partial sounds in the production of these consonants is missing or continually mispronounced the sound combination will be affected in a similar manner. Frequently we find that single parts are not affected but the combination is omitted, replaced, or mispronounced. This is not to be wondered at since a slight delay in the formation of one sound after another may mar the double consonants and induce the patient to react to the sound combination in a manner psychologically unfavorable. That is, the patient may avoid such sounds where possible.

We must consider *sound substitution* in connection with a statement in the second chapter:

> "As a rule in persons unable to achieve desired results with the usual amount of will or innervation the function completely ceases."

In this connection we will begin to appreciate why the dysarthric child, unable to produce a desired sound, does not use a similar one from the same zone of articulation, but rather jumps to a wholly different one. The most incredible sound substitutions occur on this basis. This is the reason the speech sounds of the majority of dysarthric children are more unnatural than can be explained by their brain lesion.

It is to be hoped that the opinion expressed at the beginning of this chapter will be justified; namely, that the description of isolated cases of untrained dysarthric speech is of no particular value.

The numberless variations and the changes, temporary and permanent, which may occur in the speech of a single patient substantiates the viewpoint that analytical procedure is the only one possible for orientation in the maze of dysarthric speech.

Let us now consider the method for experimental investigation of articulation. For this purpose the rubber ball with a glass tube previously described, may be used. With the rubber ball placed in the mouth the patient is instructed to repeat a con-

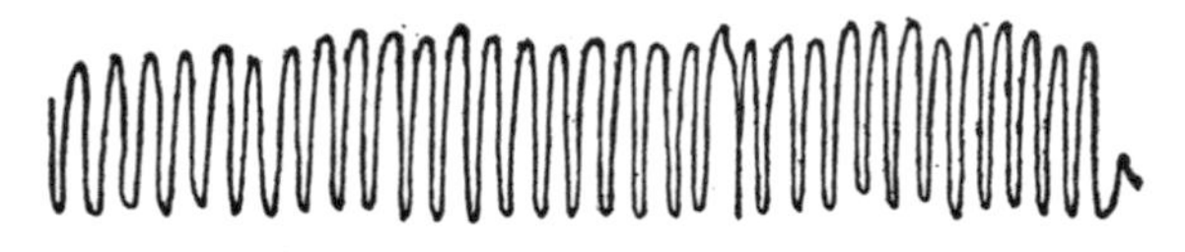

Fig. 15

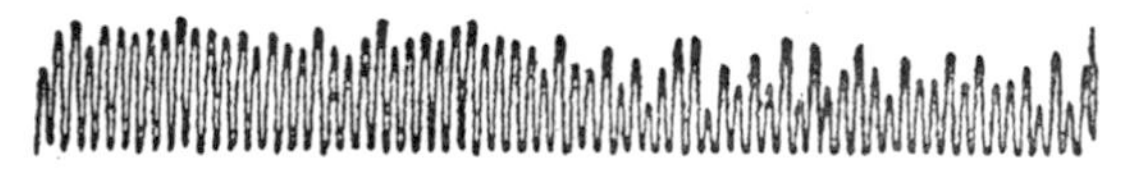

Fig. 16

sonant, a series of consonants, and then syllables. If a more complicated coordination is desired the patient may be instructed to change the vowels in the syllables. The next figures (15, 16) show the recording of the syllables "dadada" and "bababa" as spoken by a normal person. The distance between, as well as the height of, the individual peaks are uniform, almost without exception. In comparing figures 17, 18, 19 with figures 15, 16 it will be apparent that the lips and tip of the tongue of the patient (Fig. 17, 18, 19) could hardly compress the rubber ball, and the rate is highly irregular. Figs. 20, 21 are the result of four weeks'

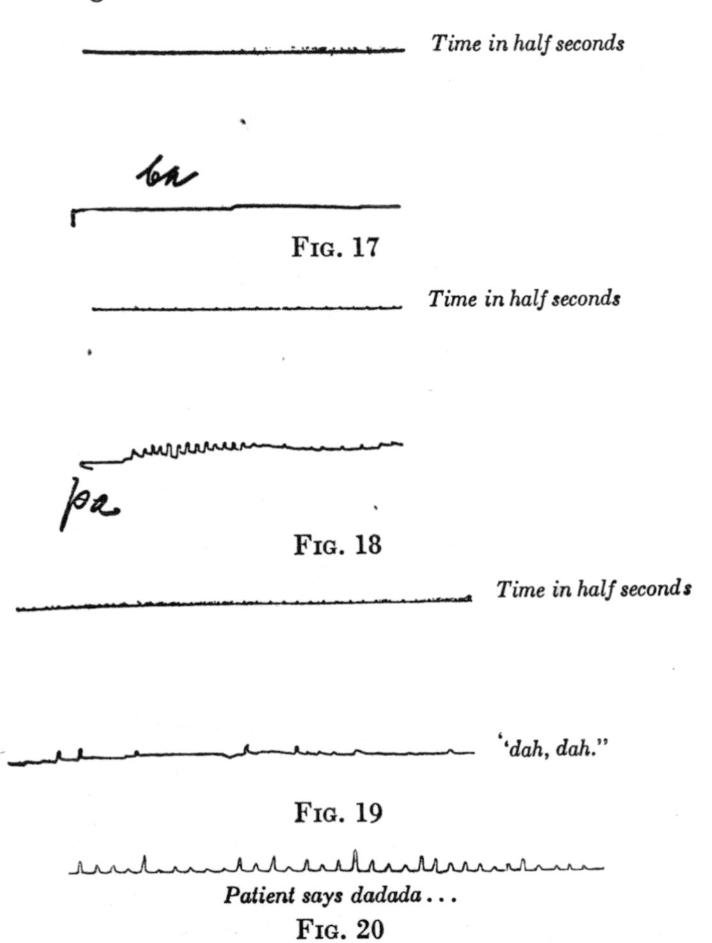

FIG. 17

FIG. 18

FIG. 19

Patient says dadada . . .

FIG. 20

treatment. The next two figures (22, 23) show the result of articulation of "pahpapeepopoo" by a normal person and the same row of vowels with T substituted for P. Now compare the figures

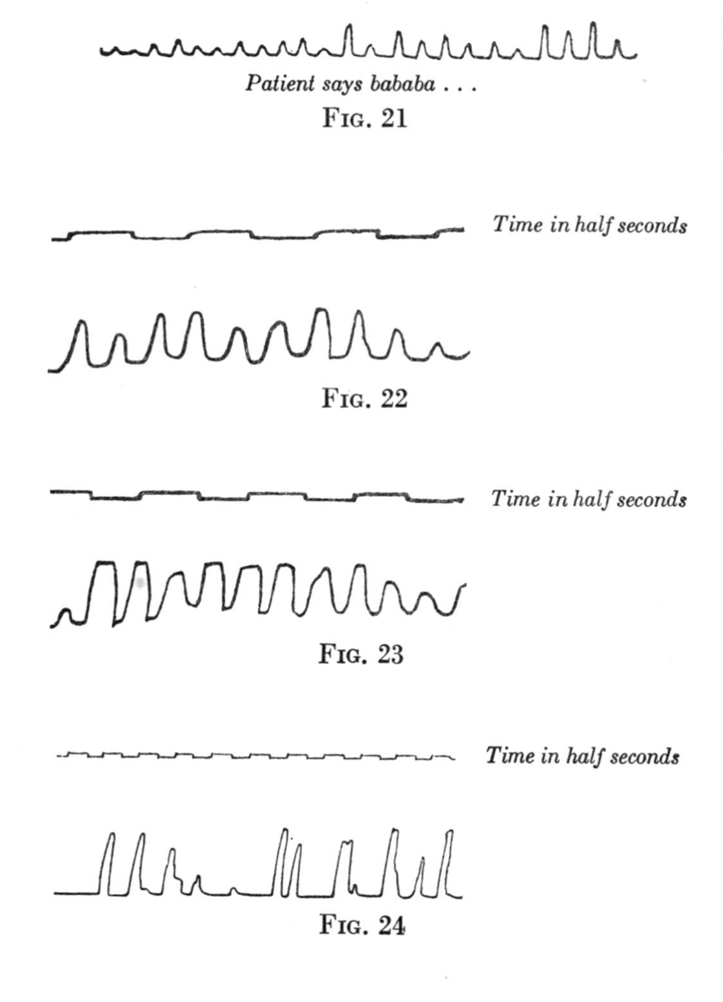

Patient says bababa . . .

FIG. 21

FIG. 22

FIG. 23

FIG. 24

22, 23, with the following graphs (Fig. 24, 25) showing the articulation curves of a dysarthric patient.*

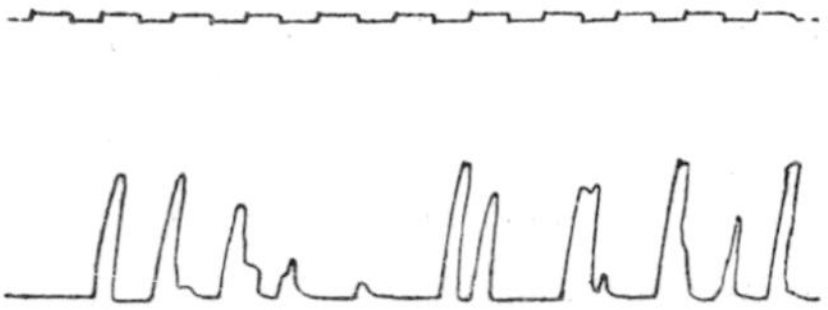

Time in half seconds

Fig. 25

*In a recent publication *Westlake* also stresses upon the necessity of analysis of the basic functions in dysarthric speech (exhaling, sustaining an even tone, opening and closing the mouth, raising the tip of the tongue, moving it from one corner of the mouth to the other, stretching the lips, peristaltic activity of the tongue). *Westlake, H.*, "Muscle Training for Cases of Cerebral Palsy." The J. of Speech and Hearing Disorders. 16, 2. June 1951, pp. 103–109.

SEVENTH CHAPTER

SIGMATISM AND RHINOLALIA

The S and SH sounds may be pathologically modified in different ways, all of which are manifest to our ears and which we may define acoustically. Unquestionably each and every sound may be distorted in varying degrees, but if any consonant, D for instance, or a vowel, is produced slightly more laterally than normal it is not so disturbing to our ear as would be the case of S or SH. The difference between S and SH on the one hand, and the rest of the consonants on the other, denotes that S and SH require a more exact pronunciation and articulation than the remaining sounds. The acute awareness of the slightest deviation in the production of S and SH sounds which have the smallest "physiological breadth" necessitates our special consideration of them apart from the other sounds, and they are designated *sigmatism.*

Sigmatisms are particularly interesting to the therapist of dysarthric speech since a defective S sound may be a minute indication of an injury to the central nervous system. Correct formation of S depends upon the very complicated coordination required of the tongue muscles. For instance, we recall that the tip of the tongue may touch, but only very slightly and elastically, the lower incisors or may approach, but must not touch, the upper incisors. We should further remember that this subtle function is joined with the formation of a groove along the median line of the tongue. It is obvious that such a delicate collaboration can easily be interfered with. Only a neurological examination can find out whether any form of sigmatism results from an organic defect or is functional in nature.

If the tongue is erroneously pressed firmly against the lower teeth the air can no longer be emitted in a jet, since it is impossible to form a groove in which the air should be gathered. A similar sound will be heard in the case of sigmatism which results from a strong pressure against the upper incisors. As a result of both these conditions the air is not released as a fine stream but in a fan-like manner. It is well to characterize this form of speech impediment as *multilocular sigmatism.*

In *interdental sigmatism* the tip of the tongue is thrust between the lower and the upper incisors. Breath can escape on both sides, or if the jaws are not firmly closed, over the whole breadth of the tongue. Most children who are afflicted with this trouble place the tongue also between the teeth in producing D, T, N, and L. We term this state *multiple interdentality.*

In *lateral sigmatism* we have a condition in which one edge of the tongue rises higher than the other, with the result that air escapes on one side only or to a greater extent on one side than on the other.

Finally there is also a *nasal sigmatism.* When the S sound is being produced normally the soft palate effects occlusion between the mouth and the nose. If this occlusion is imperfect or is totally lacking, the air will pass through the nose. This disturbance is frequently joined with a peculiar snoring sound designated as *snoring sigmatism.* (*Silbiger.*)*

Sometimes S is replaced by SH, while on the other hand, SH can be replaced by normal S or any one of the abnormal S sounds.

The *experimental methods* for diagnosis of sigmatism are numerous. We will consider only those that are not too complicated. The combination of glass and rubber tubing is an effective aid for the exact detection of the path which the air takes. The therapist will adjust the rubber tube to one end of the glass tube inserting the other end of the rubber tube into his ear, moving the small end of the glass tube around the lips of the patient from one corner of the mouth to the other while the patient emits a prolonged S sound. Carefully note the small end of the glass tube in order to detect from which point of the

*Wiener Med. Woch. 1928.

patient's mouth a definite auditive impression is derived. The therapist should make the experiment first upon himself, and he will note that the air escapes from the middle of his mouth only, while with the patient he may detect air escaping along the whole opening of the mouth. If the therapist observes that the tongue protrudes between the teeth the condition should be diagnosed as *interdental sigmatism.* If the tongue lies behind the teeth with the air escaping along the entire opening of the mouth the diagnosis should be *multilocular sigmatism.* If examination proves the air to escape on one side of the mouth only, or to a far greater extent on one side than on the other, the diagnosis of *lateral sigmatism* is justified. This form of sigmatism can also be detected by the method introduced by *Wurst* and *Fuehring.** It consists of frequent and rapid successive slight tapping with the middle finger one cheek and then the other. On the side where the air or where the main volume of air is escaping the percussion will result in interruptions of the noise produced by the air synchronically with the taps. This method is also excellent in determining SH formed unilaterally.

This is not the place to treat the question of the relation between *sigmatism* and *teeth position.*

**Fuehring, M.* and *Wurst, F.*, "Ein Beitrag zur Diagnose des Sigmatismus Lateralis." Eos, Vienna, 1930, 22, pp. 135–136.

In the book "Practice of Voice and Speech Therapy"† this question has been thoroughly discussed.

The therapy of dysarthric speech can, in the opinion of the author, only follow a treatment of the speech muscles which must be preceded by treatment of the other parts of the body. Methods for the treatment of rhinolalia and sigmatism will, therefore, be presented in a later chapter after the general therapy to induce the right coordination has been discussed.

When it can be demonstrated that in the production of *mouth sounds* a large part of the speech-air escapes through the nose, we designate this as *hyperrhinolalia.* Gross organic defects of the palate will, as a rule, induce the appearance of this speech defect, but there is a possibility that a cleft in the hard palate for example may be covered from above to such an extent by hypertrophic turbinates* that no speech defect results. Some people with this defect direct the air so skillfully that it does not get into the nose, or at least only a very small amount. The diversion of air can be shown by the usual methods of registering speech movements. *Czermak*‡ made

---

†*Froeschels* and *Jellinek*, Expression Company, Magnolia, 1941.

*The unaffected turbinates are normal bulgings at the sidewalls of the nose.

‡Ueber das Verhalten des normalen Gaumens. Sitzungsbericht der Kaiserlichen Akademie der Wissenschaften in Wien, 1887, Bd. XXIV.

use of a mirror which he held in front of the nose and which showed moisture after the enunciation of a mouth-sound if hyperrhinolalia were present. The skilled therapist will readily be able to diagnose this condition acoustically in the majority of cases if he has the patient repeat specific sounds and words. In doubtful cases *Gutzmann*‡ has the patient repeat Ah-Ee many times, frequently closing the patient's nose during the repetition. In cases where air rushes through the nose in a pathological manner it will be stopped by the obstacle, thus creating a *muffling of resonance.* In the case of normal speech this experiment is negative. It has been recommended that the diagnostician feel the nostrils of the patient during the emission of voiced sounds, as the passage of air in such cases creates a clearly perceptible vibration.

An organic as well as a functional form of *hyperrhinolalia* may be distinguished. The common organic form is caused by a pathological opening between the oral and nasal cavity in the region of the hard or the soft palate, such as a cleft in the palate, or a syphilitic aperture in the palate as a result of which the occlusion required for production of oral sounds is impossible.

Congenital cleft of the palate called "Wolfsrachen" is the result of inhibition of development

‡Untersuchungen ueber das Wesen der Nasalitaet. Archiv fuer Laryngologie und Rhinologie. 27.7. 1913.

during certain periods of embryonic growth. Normally, in the ninth embryonic week symmetric parts forming the palate coming from the sides, accrete with two intermedial bones (intermaxillaries) and these accrete with the medial part coming from the front. In the back where there is no intermaxillary, accretion of the lateral parts takes place. If only one lateral half comes into union with the intermaxillary and the latter with the medial part, a unilateral cleft occurs. If it is true of both halves a bi-lateral cleft results. There are cases also where the anterior parts unite and a fissure is left in the rear portion, or the accretion forms behind and is missing in front. (Cleft posterior or anterior respectively.)

Hyperrhinolalia occurs *also* with paralysis of the soft palate which may be either organic (as, for instance, after diphtheria or in cerebral palsy) or functional, in which case only the speech act is disturbed but not that of swallowing.

A functional trouble may also result from paralyzed muscles which normally collaborate with the soft palate in the production of speech. At this time, it is well to mention that there have been cases of cerebral palsy with hyperrhinolalia functionalis in which treatment of the paralyzed lips and the paralyzed tongue resulted not only in strengthening these muscles but also in improvement of the palatal function. One such case will be found described in Chapter X.

In every hyperrhinolalia in which no cleft palate is evident the hard palate must be examined along its medial line; many times there is felt at the border between the hard and the soft palate a defect in the bone of the former. Here at the posterior border of the hard palate is the place of insertion of the muscles of the soft palate. Now it is clear that defects in the hard palate will diminish the possibility of muscle insertion. If the space for muscle insertion is too small the soft palate cannot be supposed to function normally. We must not overlook the fact that also defects throughout the length of the hard palate are frequently covered by a normal appearing mucous membrane so that they are invisible to the eye.

Opposite to hyperrhinolalia we have the speech defect characterized by a deficiency of resonance called *hyporhinolalia.* In this case we may again have an organic or a functional basis. Proliferation in the nose and in the upper pharynx, for instance, the well known enlargement of the nasopharyngeal tonsil "adenoid", deviations of the nasal septum, swelling of the turbinates, etc., in part prevent resonance in the nose when the nasal sounds M, N and NG are being formed.* When voiced oral sounds are formed the air in the nose vibrates also as an effect of the percussion of the

*Since vowels directly preceding or following a nose-sound, also to a smaller extent are nasalized physiologically, they will be affected too by hyporhinolalia.

hard palate which results from vibrations in the oral cavity. Therefore, disturbances of nasal resonance will also be present in these sounds. An analogous auditive impression will result from defective movements in certain muscles of the pharynx, especially in cramps or cramp-like conditions of the soft palate, which, as we know, are frequently signs of dysarthria.

There is a third form of rhinolalia called *mixed rhinolalia.* This clinical picture occurs in cases of a pathological communication between mouth and nose if adenoids or other deformities prevent the air from vibrating in the nose during the pronunciation of M, N, Ng.

Eighth Chapter

GENERAL THERAPY TO INDUCE CO-ORDINATION AND CONTROL OF VOLUNTARY MUSCLES

Fundamentally there are several ways available for testing whatever muscle group we intend to test, a weak or a tense, an athetoid, an atactic or a trembling one. Under normal conditions striped (voluntary) muscles acquire their skill to function under the influence of centripetal sensory impressions, seeing, hearing, etc. (leading to the centers) and under the influence of centrifugal stimulations (deriving and going into the body from the centers). In Chapter III the acquisition of the skill of speaking was analyzed according to the centripetal and centrifugal influences. We need not deal here with cases in which only a centripetal function is wanting (*f.i.* in congenitally deaf children), but with those in which either one or more centrifugal functions are wanting, (*e.g.* with a case in which the transmission of motor impulses from the anterior central convolution into the muscles of the leg or the mouth is hindered) or in which exists in addition a hardness of hearing or a lack of feeling of the movements performed (due to a lesion of the pathways from the muscles to the posterior central convolution).

As pointed out in Chapter IX therapy must aim at strengthening of weakened muscles and/or at reducing the degree of contraction, eliminating, as far as possible, athetoid movements and tremor, and improving atactic conditions.

Unless one can successfully use drugs, massage, bathing, electricity, etc., the ways available are chiefly sensory. In some cases optic control of the athetoid movements (*e.g.* looking at the athetoid hand or looking at the face in a mirror) or of the muscles which are in a state of tremor is helpful. In other cases or in those mentioned above the acoustic impressions received from the speech therapist may improve the patient's speech, especially if he executes acoustic and visual control of his own speech, such as comparing the impressions coming from the mouth of the therapist with those coming from his own speech. Tactile sensory impressions are frequently of great influence. This is true especially in cases in which the sense of touch and/or the sensory impressions deriving from muscles and periosteum are weak because of disturbances within the centripetal nerves or the receptive center. Some patients must touch certain parts of their mouths (*e.g.* the lips, the tip or the back of the tongue, the soft palate) to get an idea of their position and/or of the movements they perform. Tactile control of the chest wall and the anterior abdominal wall in breathing may also be necessary. The stiffness of overcontracted muscles escapes the notice of most of the spastics until they are taught to touch them. It is very important to inform the patient in the same way about the different conditions of such muscles after they have been brought into a more relaxed state. One would not assume that many patients need tactile control to become fully aware of the jerking movements of their athetoid muscles. But experience proves that this is the case. They are surprised about the extent to which those muscles move involuntarily. Optic *and* tactile control will work still more effectively.

If we ask ourselves why many patients are not fully aware of their abnormal movements there are several possible explanations. The centripetal impressions may be weak. But in every case the forming of habit patterns is also a reason. Under normal conditions habits also often escape full awareness. It is therefore the therapist's aim to lift these abnormal habit patterns into the conscious mind of the patient. *Rutherford** offers a scheme for the treatment of habit patterns. The patient must first learn to identify them by looking into a mirror, in other words, to become aware of what he does if he for example lifts an arm, starts

---

*l. c.

talking, etc. Then he should recognize the movements without help of a mirror, just kinesthetically. He should be guided to understand the probable original use of each pattern of movements. By optic or tactile control the patient should find out "how he does it". He should study all parts of the pattern. The clinician should touch various points in the area of movements, asking each time, "Do you feel it here?" The next step consists of voluntary imitation of the pathological habitual movement, also of those observed in other patients. Finally the patient should learn to eliminate the habit pattern by relaxation. The newly acquired movements that should be as close as possible to norm must be trained again and again by voluntary innervations until they become a habit.

Which sensory impressions are used during a treatment depends upon the single clinical picture. There is not a rigid schedule; on the contrary shifting from one sense to the other may prove necessary in every moment.

Reflexes may also be used to develop voluntary movements. The gag reflex can be initiated and the patient may learn in this way to widen the pharynx and to drop the back of the tongue (two movements which may be useful in correcting faulty pronunciation of vowels). In some patients this reflex cannot be provoked because of paralysis of the respective neurons. Strong stimulations such as strong pressure against the back of the tongue, the pharyngeal wall or light touching of the fauces may still provoke a reflex and in this way the reflex may gradually become "canalized". If the gag reflex is too strong, which is rarely the case, one may succeed in diminishing it also by provoking it frequently. Speaking of reflexes, it must be mentioned that swallowing often is performed with great difficulty. Here also the therapist may try to "canalize" the reflex by first moving a morsel slowly from the lips over the tongue to the pharynx. Then the patient can stimulate it by using his own finger.

The difficulties mentioned so far to be encountered by the therapist and the patient are in every case complicated by psychogenic symptoms (See page 161). To encourage the patient, to correct him in a friendly manner, even to avoid correcting him at times are some of the ways to eliminate fatigue, depression, and stubbornness. The right psychological attitude on the part of the therapist is no less decisive for a final success than his technical knowledge, skill and experience.

When and how should treatment of dysarthria begin? When should general treatment begin and when special treatment? There is only one answer: As early as possible. When the diagnosis of dysarthria is made, followed by differential diagnosis between organic and functional spasticity, if athetoid movements, ataxia and tremor, have been recognized immediate treatment should be instituted. A neurologist and physiotherapist will not hesitate to use electricity and massage even on a suckling. They will recommend later on special devices (chair, walker) adjusted to the special needs of the case, and will advise the use of some gymnastic apparatus. Generally speaking, a muscle-strengthening treatment can be developed to a certain degree without the patient's co-operation. However, another treatment is imperative in many cases, a treatment which aims at relaxation. It cannot begin before the child understands relatively complicated instructions and is willing to obey them. Advanced therapeutic methods requiring imitative exercises demonstrated by the therapist demand also the willingness of the child to co-operate. The age at which these two phases of physiotherapy may begin must be determined in each individual case.

We cannot undertake here to describe and outline an entire comprehensive treatment of the voluntary muscles of the body in cases of spastic or flabby paralysis. There are many reasons for such restriction. In the first place, general treatment is a matter for determination by the family doctor, the pediatrist, the neurologist, the physiotherapist and the surgeon. We dedicate this work to the speech therapists, to parents, and to those in care of spastic children. General musculature treatment calls for no less differential diagnostic work than does special treatment of the voice and speech of these patients. The differential diagnosis concerning muscles not participating in production of voice and speech belongs to the neurologist and not to the speech therapist. The neurologist and the other physicians mentioned above may gradually instruct the mother and those in charge of dysarthric cases, but this specific skill cannot be gained from books any more than the neurologist could replace the speech therapist through analogous study. The speech therapist may instruct and introduce the parents and attendants in his special work. However, no one must expect that a study of this volume will give the expertness necessary to treat the speech of the dysarthric child without the supervision of a speech therapist. One of the greatest mistakes a layman can make is to use an exercise excessively or to prolong its application when it is no longer required. Here also only the therapist can give the correct instructions.

Refraining from describing a therapy for musculature in general, nevertheless we must give some suggestions for such treatment. This is necessitated by the references that have been made to "general relaxation" in discussing speech therapy. Now, an explanation of "general relaxation" is required for an adequate understanding of dysarthric speech therapy. That general muscle training is absolutely necessary before and during speech treatment is obvious from the considerations made thus far.* We have learned that spastic muscles may influence unfavorably other remote muscles, and that surrounding paretic muscles may hinder more or less a normal muscle in its function. In addition, the patient's consciousness of being handicapped in some part of the body may influence his attitude adversely against any kind of movement. Experience proves that relaxation of spastic, highly contracted and tense muscles in other parts of the body will help to relax the speech muscles. (*Pusitz*,† *O'Brien*.‡)

Another reason why it is impossible for the speech therapist to refrain from dealing with general musculature treatment is that he is concerned with a function essential for speech, life and movement as well — namely, respiration. Respiration is a matter of major consideration in dysarthric speech, since it is frequently affected in such states. Constituting the source of disturbed speech and voice (in a certain sense) defective respiration must be corrected in order to improve speech and voice. When we note the fact that more than half the body participates in the movements of

*See also: *Carroll, Robert L.*, "Speech Training in the Child Crippled by Spastic Paralysis." J. Speech Disorders, 1937, 2. pp. 155–157.

†*Pusitz, M. E.*, "Speech Correction in Cerebral Palsy." J. Speech Disorders, 4, 3, Sept. 1939.

‡*O'Brien, V.*, "Treatment of Children with Cerebral Palsy." N. Y. State J. of Med., July 15, 1945, pp. 1548–1550.

respiration we realize that no part of this large area of the body can be totally eliminated from our consideration. "Probably the easiest procedure after relaxation has been . . . attempted, is to try to improve breathing," writes *Evans*.§

Naturally the greatest relaxation of muscles and muscle-groups is best attained by cessation of all activity — complete rest. For this reason the patient should begin relaxation training in a position on the back (supine). In many cases this position is most helpful in establishing the abdominal movements which accompany diaphragmatic breathing and for training the patient in improving this type of respiration. When he lies on his back expansion of the chest is restricted to some extent which results in vicariously stronger action of the diaphragm. The entire abdominal wall will rise remarkably during inhaling while the patient is reclining on the back. The hands of the child should be placed on the abdominal wall that he may sense the lifting and lowering which accompanies inhalation and exhalation. A firm fixation of these "conditions" characterizing diaphragmatic breathing—namely, strong inward and outward movements, if carried over into an upright position, will tend to strengthen diaphragmatic breathing and cause the dysarthric to use it. The practice of diaphragmatic breathing exercises

§*Evans, Marsee Fred,* "Problems in Cerebral Palsy." J. Speech Disorders, 1947, 12, pp. 87–103.

when standing offers an opportunity for training the patient also in correct thoracic breathing, since in normal individuals and in most of those with pathological conditions, both types of respiration are present. The upright position favors establishment and tactile control of the synchronous movements of the chest wall and the forward and backward movement of the anterior abdominal wall. The patient should be taught to strengthen thoracic breathing when it is weak even if there is no pathological incongruity between thoracic and abdominal breathing. To accomplish this he should receive visual and tactile impressions through the use of a large mirror with his hands placed on his chest. It is well to accompany strong inhalation and exhalation with synchronic up-and-downward movements of the arms, not higher than the height of the shoulders and other movements of the arms as a means of enlarging the chest. See Figs. 26, 27, 28.

In cerebral or spinal cord palsy one half of the chest may move less than the other half*; hence, calling the visual and tactile senses into play is frequently not enough to bring about adequate respiratory movements of the more seriously

---

**Samzelius-Lejdstroem* has described a preponderance of the right half of the chest over the left as a physiological appearance. (Sixth meeting of the International Society for Logopedy and Phoniatry. Copenhagen, 1936. Publisher: Deuticke, Vienna and Leipzig. Pathologically the difference in the respiratory movements may be extremely large.

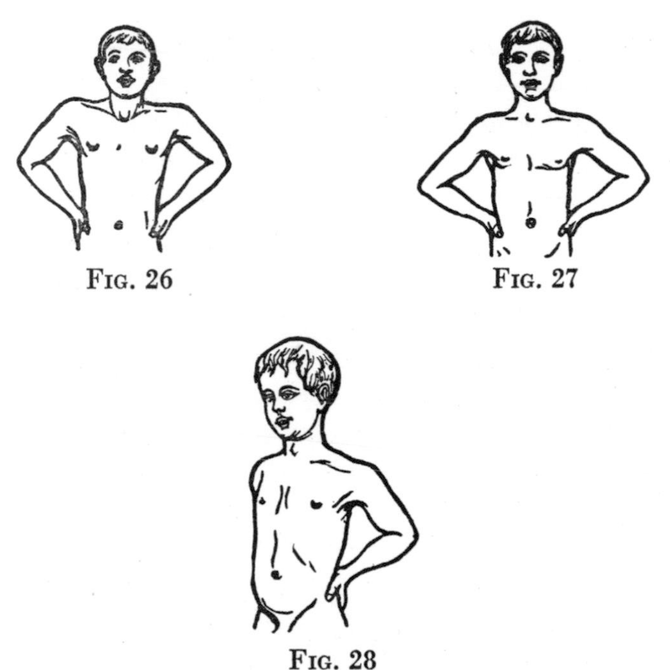

Fig. 26

Fig. 27

Fig. 28

(From: Schreber's "Zimmer Gymnastik.")

affected side. But here physiology offers us resources, as there exists an amazing relationship between half of the nose and the corresponding half of the chest. If you close one nostril and inhale through the other with closed mouth, you will feel that part of the chest corresponding to the closed nostril answer immediately with feeble respiratory movement, while the movement of the other side becomes stronger. We can exploit this observation for treatment of such cases. By having the patient breathe only through the nostril on the more affected side while closing the other, we will induce stronger movements of the corresponding side of the thorax. *All respiratory exercises should be practiced at least ten times a day but for not more than a minute's duration.* In this instance, as in all other exercises of the body and speech muscles with dysarthrics, a definite limit may be set for our therapeutic efforts.

If the patient inhales through the mouth, it should be silently, since accompanying noise indicates a glottis that is too narrow due to a functional or organic spasm of the closers on the one hand, or flabbiness of the openers on the other. Another cause of such noise may be retraction of the tongue toward the pharynx. In the latter case, the patient must be taught to touch his under incisors with the tip of the tongue. Sometimes nose- as well as mouth-breathing must be trained. The first by closing the mouth, the latter by opening it. *Rutherford's** modified spirometer seems to be a good help for this kind of training. The use of pinwheels and soap bubbles is advisable in many cases.

Sometimes, especially in little children, the therapist should use rhythmical pressure on the lower ribs while the patient lies in prone position. In this way he may acquire the feeling for rhythmical breathing which is missing in some dysarthrics.

**Rutherford, Berneice R.*: "Give Them a Chance to Talk." Burgess Publ. Comp., Minneapolis, Minnesota, 1948.

The reader may gain the impression that our plan first to introduce methods of general relaxation has been abandoned, but we should keep in mind that any method aiming at securing relaxation must take breathing into account. Breathing exercises are of the greatest importance in the establishment of relaxation. It is necessary, therefore, to introduce relaxation through training in breathing exercises.† It will depend on the conditions in each individual case whether only a few of such exercises should be given in each series as introduction to relaxation, or whether a more extensive training of respiration should be made before beginning attempts at securing relaxation.

In turning to special exercises in *relaxation* we begin the work by having the patient assume a supine position (on his back). He is instructed to close his eyes and to imagine he is asleep. The following may be suggested to him: "You are lying in a meadow basking in warm sunshine. The air is cool and the soft breeze moves over your body. You dream that you are moved about by the breeze. Your body has no weight. Everything is perfectly relaxed and there is no tautness. Your head is wafted toward the left, since your neck is soft and pliable. You raise your right arm but the breeze blows it down since it too is lissom, as are the legs and the other

---

†*Roon, Karin* (Report of Classes in Applied Relaxation. Copyright by K. Roon) also emphasizes the close relationship between relaxation and breathing exercises.

arm. The breeze changes its direction and blows your head to the right. All of this is very pleasing to you and you do not feel any resistance in your body to the soft breeze." Have the child open his eyes and imitate the flabby movements of his neck and limbs. Direct him to turn on his stomach and repeat the exercises in this position. Similar expedients may be given by the therapist who, understanding the meaning of such exercises, will invent new games and devices aiming at the same purpose.

Relaxation exercises may also be prescribed for the child in the form of games. *Barrows* and *Hall** recommend playing "rag doll." Such rag dolls have no stiff parts. An arm elevated will fall down if released. The head will fall forward or backward or sideward if not fixed by someone. Ask the child to imitate this flabbiness and you will stimulate him to relaxation. Older children may profit also by the use of games for strengthening as well as for relaxation.

Relaxation must be striven for in every possible position — sitting, standing, walking. Those exercises which have as their aim *strengthening of the muscles* are so well known that their description can be omitted; in addition, the speech specialist is not concerned to a great extent with their use. It is well to mention here an expedient known

**Barrows* and *Hall*, "Jack in the Box." Expression Company, Magnolia, Massachusetts.

to the neurologist and speech therapist which we will exemplify in the case of a paralyzed tongue. It may be encouraging for the therapist to learn that in the cases in question, glossoplegia could often be improved. A spatula was placed under the tongue elevating the organ with the *slightest force necessary* while directing the patient to assist by spontaneous raising of the tongue. In other words, *from the beginning the passive movement is accompanied by active intention.* This combining of passive and active movements is necessary in any kind of muscle strengthening treatment (*e.g.* jaw, lips). At the beginning it is a difficult task for both patient and therapist, but if they persevere in it they will be rewarded by success.

The *Bobaths** have also made thorough studies about the mutual influence of sometimes far distant muscles on other muscles and have made use of these studies in therapy. Spasticity of an arm may be diminished by having the legs flexed maximally at the hips and knee, or arms flexed if legs are treated. The publication of the *Bobaths* deserves, in the author's opinion, thorough reading.

Athetoid and choreatic movements can be diminished by careful visual observation of the parts affected. If, for instance, one hand is affected instruct the child to stretch his fingers widely and bring them together again slowly and carefully,

---

**Bobath, K.* and *Bobath, B.*, "Spastic Paralysis." The British J. of Physical Medicine, June, 1950.

observing them all the while. Next ask him to keep the fingers as still and passive as possible, meanwhile observing them. It is difficult and at times impossible at first to avoid a violent stiffening of the arm muscles during this drill.

Optimum contraction must be sought in order to prevent active spasticity. The result of treating choreatic and athetoid movements seems to depend, at least in part, on the duration of the ailment. In several cases of patients from three to six years of age the author has succeeded in eliminating these movements entirely. This is a *prima facie* evidence that treatment should begin as early as possible. Explanation of the elimination of such movements is difficult, but it is to be supposed that those pathological movements may become automatic, much as voluntary movements do when they are permitted to extend over a period of time. This statement may appear to be contradictory to the common and accepted meaning of the word "automatic", which is generally applied to voluntary movements only, but if we consider for instance, how constipation, a malfunction of the bowels, becomes progressively worse if not treated in time, we are justified in supposing that wholly involuntary movements may become "fixed" in a similar way as voluntary movements if they are allowed to persist for a long interval.

It is a delicate point how best to use normal children as examples to aid the dysarthric patient. Only observation of the individual case can show us whether such examples work favorably as a stimulant, or unfavorably, depressing the handicapped child. Everything that may produce an inferiority complex must be avoided if possible!

Let us remember that it is the task of the neurologist and the therapist to prescribe in detail the exercises aimed at alleviation of spasticity, palsy and chorea-athetosis. Only a thorough investigation and diagnosis can be effective as a basis for treatment.

Finally, a few words about drug therapy and brain surgery. Prostigmine and neostigmine used under strict neurological indication may diminish spasticity, but not choreatic-athetoid conditions. The latter seem to react favorably upon dilantin sodium and paramit.† For hypoarthria *Wilder*‡ recommends scopolamine. No remarkable success has been achieved with any of these drugs. Therefore, the training methods are still of decisive importance.

Not much can be said nor is much known about the effect of brain surgery upon spasms, athetoid movements, atactic signs and tremor. Yet, in the progress of that branch of medicine lies, in the opinion of the author, the greatest hope for the cerebral palsy cases.§

---

†*Hartmann K.*, 59th Meeting Société Suisse de Neurologie, Dec. 1946.

‡*Wilder, J.* "Neurological Speech Disorders." New York Society for Speech and Voice Therapy, May 9, 1951.

§See, e.g.: *Browder, E. J.*: "Modification of Spastic Hemiplegia by Cortical Excision" and *Putnam's* important discussion, N. Y. Academy of Medicine, Section of Neurology and Psychiatry, Feb. 9, 1943. Archives of Neurology and Psychiatry, Sept. 1943, 50, 3, p. 367.

Ninth Chapter

SPEECH-MUSCLES TRAINING IN DYSARTHRIA

If we were asked the most valuable advice we could give for the speech treatment of spastic children the answer would be: "*Speech exercises should not begin before the best possible balance of the muscles involved has been obtained.*" Of course, in many cases the speech act can not be eliminated until this desired muscular balance is obtained as the family has encouraged the child to speak spontaneously. *This is unfortunate since defective spontaneous speech interferes with therapeutic efforts.* Let us take an example and determine what happens when a child spontaneously speaks for instance D, with a tongue which is "partly spastic". Exact diagnosis, as has been shown, very often reveals that some muscle *fibres* in dysarthria of the speech mechanism are affected in a different manner or to a different degree than other muscle fibres in the same organ. That is to say, some fibres may be normal while others are paralyzed; some may be normal while others are spastic, etc. Now, when compared with the normal state, there exists a definite interference between these differently affected parts. Those that are less paralyzed must drag or pull along the weaker ones, and the former may be handicapped in their normal strengthening and development by their paralyzed mates. Another result of this situation may be that the stronger or the unaffected parts develop a state of active spasm. It is as improbable that the weaker parts thus will be strengthened as it is to assume that the legs of a child are benefited if he is always carried about instead of being permitted or forced to walk. Furthermore, a spastic group of muscle fibres may suppress or thwart every attempt of a weaker or normal part to function at all. If the neglected choreatic movements interfere with the efforts to elevate the tongue there may result functional palsy or functional spasms of those parts not affected by chorea. We therefore may obtain unfavorable results if we begin our work with speech exercises without previous training of the muscles for a workable balance.

We must not underrate the difficulties faced by the therapist in view of the fact that the family is eager and anxious to detect speech improvement in the dysarthric child. Nevertheless, the conscientious therapist may work for several months on the muscles only. The aim is to help the child, and the hopes and desires of the family can only be fulfilled in what may seem to them to be a roundabout way. We now offer some simple methods to improve the balance between differently affected *speech muscles.*

The experience that relaxation of some muscles aids in relaxation of other parts applies also to the relaxing methods used in special speech therapy.* Therefore, they will not be discussed in relation to one part of the three-fold functions, breathing, voice production and articulation, but rather to the complete speech act. In many instances a relaxation method designed for specific speech and voice therapy will apply to the whole body. There are two relaxing techniques which must be stressed here: *jaw-shaking* and the *chewing method.*

Jaw-shaking can be described as a rapid motion of the lower jaw to both sides. The muscles which draw the jaw to the right and to the left are the pterygoid muscles. These movements should be taught in front of a mirror. The therapist should learn jaw-shaking in order to demonstrate it correctly to the patient. The exercises begin with a slow but forceful movement of the dropped jaw to both sides. With some individuals, especially with spastics, the pterygoid muscles are not accustomed to function and the joint between the under jaw and the temporal bone is stiff. This is often not a permanent but only a temporary obstacle requiring a longer period of training. Many patients learn the slow movements in one or two

*See: *Stinchfield-Hawk, Sara*: "Speech Therapy for the Physically Handicapped." Stanford University Press, Stanford, California, 1950.

days, exercising for one minute duration ten times a day. Slight pains may result but they will disappear in a short time. The rate of the shaking movements should gradually be increased until the jaw moves like a pendulum at the rate of three or four times in a second.

The idea underlying these exercises is as follows: Some superficial neck muscles are fixed along the under border of the lower jaw. Therefore shaking is possible only if these muscles are relaxed. On the other hand, shaking within itself aids these muscles to relax. Experience has shown that there exists a functional relationship between the superficial and the deeper muscles of the throat, and even of the muscles closing the glottis and stretching the vocal cords. This therapy was first introduced for the treatment of voice defects resulting from over-exertion of the laryngeal and pharyngeal muscles. The relaxing influence of jaw-shaking on these muscles became evident, whereupon they were used with dysarthric patients. Jaw-shaking later may be joined with voice production. At the beginning of the training no phonation should take place in order that the patient's attention may be concentrated solely on relaxing the muscles involved. Of course, there are cases of severe stiffness of the jaw in which shaking can only be learned after a long time, if ever.

The *chewing method* was also devised and introduced by the author for the relaxation of the voice and speech muscles (against functional hoarseness, loss of voice, stuttering, speech correction of deaf children, correction of the voice of individuals becoming hard of hearing in advanced age*). The method and technique based on various anatomical, physiological, pathological and folk psychological observations proved to be very effective in various hypertonic conditions. Experiences of everyday life make it evident that chewing, on the one hand, and speaking and singing on the other, not only have a common source, but are, *basically* one and the same function. We can speak or sing and chew food *without interrupting any one of these functions.* The chewing muscles and the muscles moving the mouth during speech and voice production are entirely identical. Different work can not be done with one and the same muscle group simultaneously. The logical conclusion must be that chewing, speaking and singing are *not different acts but one identical act.* Age-old experience teaches us that people overstrain their mouths and pharyngeal muscles in speaking and singing but never in eating. Such disorders as functional hoarseness, stuttering, etc., are in part or wholly the result of over-exertion. In the chewing exercises, the patient is directed to make chewing movements and later the chewing movements are combined with voice produc-

---

Weiss, D. and *Beebe, H.:* "The Chewing Approach in Speech and Voice Therapy." Karger, Basel. New York, 1950.

tion. The patient should "chew his voice". Care must be taken not to produce stereotyped *ngan-ganga, mamama, hamhamham*, etc., but *to really assume the psychical attitude of chewing*. The chewing should be performed simultaneously with the opening and closing of the lips. In this way, a marked improvement can be achieved. With dysarthric patients who have chewing difficulties, the spasms, as a rule, are more severe in speaking than in chewing.

This method, together with that of jaw-shaking in speech correction, should be used in accordance with our guiding idea: to teach relaxation before teaching speech. Two very remarkable experiences will illustrate the relaxing influence of the chewing movements on different parts of the body. One of these experiences came from *Dr. Hollingsworth*, the other from a former assistant of the author in Vienna, *Mrs. Schmitz-Svevo*. *Hollingsworth** published some results of his investigations of the influence of chewing on working muscles: "Without exception, with both workers and during all three kinds of work, muscular tension is decreased during the chewing period. It may well enough be that chewing as a conditioned stimulus brings with it . . . a posture of relaxation." *Mrs. Schmitz-Svevo* states:†

*"Science," 90 No. 2339.

†Paper not yet published.

"The following case of spastic paralysis, due to birth trauma, which was favorably influenced by the practice of the chewing method, seems worthy of notice. The patient, a boy of twelve, was unable to move about except on all fours, crawling on his knees with the aid of his clenched fists. He was very intelligent and was a good pupil, but he had to dictate his compositions because he was unable to hold a pen or pencil. He suffered greatly from athetoid movements and he would beat his chest for minutes at a time. Cerebral dysarthria was not present but he could produce words only in jerks probably due to a cerebellar lesion.

I explained and demonstrated the chewing method to this bright boy and soon, by means of it, he was able to speak smoothly, though more slowly than a normal person does. As he went through his exercises, I realized how effective, in general, was the chewing method in his case. The cramped fingers relaxed sufficiently to enable him to hold and also to pick up corks of various sizes; eventually he could also move a pencil across the page. The chewing method enabled him to acquire relaxation before my eyes. Attempts to stand on his braced legs and to take a few steps proved successful. After some time, he could be led from his work-table to the window, a distance of about three meters. There he would remain standing and watch the children playing in the street. The therapy for this patient required six weeks, following which his mother took over the work with him."

Perlstein and *Shere** also recommend the Chewing Method for dysarthric speech and *Gratke*† deals with the improvement of chewing. *Sittig*‡ reports on the cessation of excessive salivation and drooling in cerebral palsy. *Kastein*§ used the Chewing Method successfully in non-athetoid cases. With these patients she introduced a treatment that is based on the principle of establishing resistance "in order to bring into play the automatic enervation of all muscles concerned. At the present stage an elastic bandage is used and tied around the head, mask like, covering the temples, cheeks and chin and allowing just enough freedom of motion to enable the patient to move his jaw and chin downward against the pull of the bandage, during articulation." The author has no personal experience with this new method but has seen good results when the Chewing Method

---

**M. A. Perlstein* and *M. Shere*. "Speech Therapy in Children with Cerebral Palsy." Am. Journ. of Diseases of Children. 72, Oct. 1946, p. 389.

†*J. M. Gratke*. "Speech Problems of the Cerebral Palsied." Journ. of Speech Disorders. 12. 2. June 1947. pp. 129–134.

‡*E. Sittig*. "The Chewing Method Applied for Excessive Salivation and Drooling in Cerebral Palsy." Journ. of Speech Disorders. 12, 2. June 1947. p. 191.

§*S. Kastein*. "Speech Therapy in Cerebral Palsy." Journal of Rehabilitation. June 1948.

was used also in the athetoid type. *Palmer*,* after careful studies of the function of the mandible, recommends chewing after having, if necessary, brought forth some inhibition by gently touching the hyperactive muscles and moving the jaw up and down.

The explanation of why chewing helps speech in cerebral palsy lies at least partly in the fact that chewing is less "emotionally burdened" than speaking because chewing does not involve social obligations. Therefore by shifting from the idea and attitude of speaking to that of chewing the social factors are eliminated. This explanation is in line with the findings of *Heltman* and *Peacher*† which point to a psychological factor involved in dysarthrias. It seems that *Robbins*‡ is very close to the Chewing Method when he asks the patient to make faces before a mirror, to sigh aloud, without allowing any muscle to stop moving or to become tense.

As has been mentioned above, the tongue paralyzed on one side or paralyzed to a greater degree on one side than on the other deviates to the

---

**F. M. Palmer*. "Studies in Clinical Techniques. Mandibular Facet Slip in Cerebral Palsy." Journ. of Speech Disorders. 1, 13. March 1948. pp. 44–48.

†*H. J. Heltman* and *G. M. Peacher*. "Misarticulation and Diadokokinesis in Spastic Paralytic." Journ. of Speech Disorders. 8. 2. June 1943. pp. 137–145.

‡*S. D. Robbins*. "Dysarthria and its Treatment." Journ. of Speech Disorders. V, 2. June 1940. pp. 113–120.

weaker side. This fact deserves to be considered. If a patient with this condition desires to produce a sound in the second zone of articulation as D, T, N, L, SH, he must elevate the tip of the tongue. In this attempt, the weaker, as well as the stronger portions, will mutually hinder one another. The stronger part by deviating will have difficulty in approaching the upper middle incisor teeth, while the action of the weaker portion is almost completely eliminated. No wonder this strain stimulates other easily excitable muscles to involuntary collaboration. The muscles of the face are especially conditioned for such participation which seems to be one reason why ugly grimaces appear in some dysarthric children. In some cases, the grimaces appear only upon the pronunciation of sounds in the second zone of articulation and seem to be limited to the muscular co-ordination required for the production of such sounds. In other cases, the grimaces, though weaker, are also present when other sounds are produced. This may, however, be only the result of habit. Whether or not this explanation covers all the factors involved, at least the attempt to bring into muscular balance both sides of the tongue has sometimes proved a most successful expedient. The experiment of moving the tongue with a spatula and holding it toward the weaker side *resulted in the immediate cessation of grimacing.* Dysarthric patients could readily repeat this procedure themselves and could practice relaxing the stronger part of the tongue so that any deviation would become less marked or even disappear with accompanying improvement of the facial expression. The following two figures (Fig. 29 and 30) show a boy of sixteen years

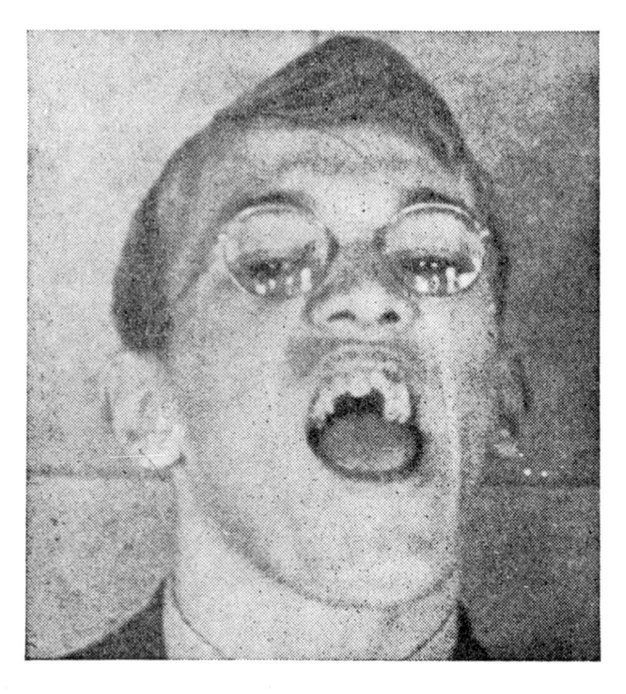

FIG. 29

saying "ah" before, and ten days after the beginning of treatment. No grimaces are present in the second photograph.

Of the methods employed for the *strengthening of the paralyzed muscles*, pushing of the arms will be described in Chapter XI. Electric treatment and massage of the soft palate will also be considered in Chapter XI.

To strengthen the muscles of the lips, the author used several bottle corks of different sizes, each

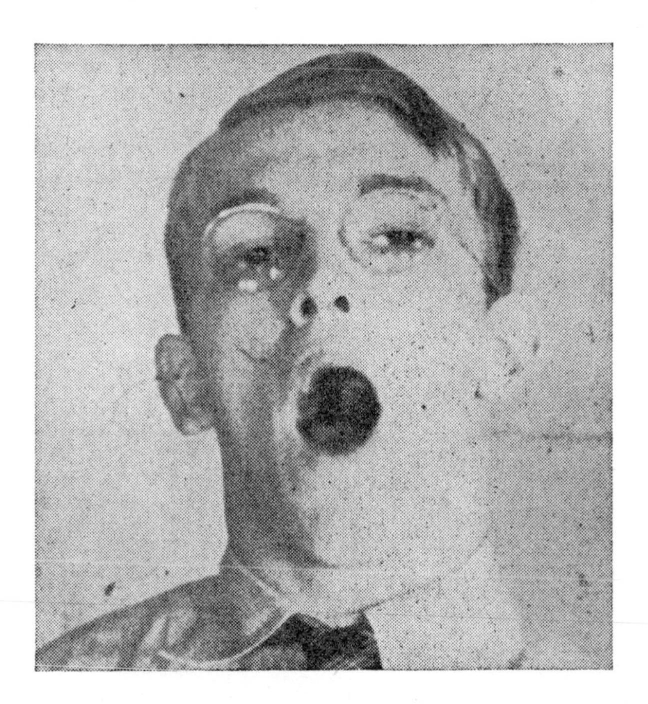

FIG. 30

of them one mm larger in diameter than the next size. The smallest in the series had a diameter of one cm, the largest three cm. The patient was directed to hold the corks one after another with his lips but not to bite them, thus eliminating the aid of the jaw muscles. On this occasion, a strange observation was made. With few exceptions, the patients could hold and retain some of the corks between the lips but could not hold or retain others. This would not be so noteworthy if there had been a great difference in the diameter of the corks which could be held and those which could not be held. There was, however, a striking difference in the function of the lip muscles with the corks differing only one mm. That certainly indicates that some muscle fibres were more affected by paralysis than others, and hence, these findings are of great importance. Let us assume that a therapist employs only one object, for instance, a pencil one cm in diameter, to ascertain the strength of the lip muscles of the patient. Now, if a patient is able to hold the pencil with his lips, it may be assumed that he does not suffer from palsy of the lips. *In reality, only those fibres of the lip muscles the contraction of which results in an opening of one cm were tested with this experiment.* It is therefore necessary that a complete examination should be made. The corks should also be used as an exercise designed to strengthen the weak fibres of the lip muscles and if they are gradually employed, good results will be effected.

Training in rhythm is most important because rhythmical movements can only be executed well when there exists a state of balance between protagonists and antagonists and voluntary rapid rhythmical movements are possible only if both of these muscles are neither spastic nor paralytic. In addition, we must keep in mind that speech has a pronounced rhythmical component, the slightest impairment of which immediately interferes with the speech act. It is a commonplace observation that rapid movements are normally more easily executed with rhythm. An individual can raise and drop his index finger or his jaw in such a way that rhythm is absent but if the speed is gradually increased, a point will eventually be reached beyond which it would be impossible to prevent rhythm from entering and governing the act. Therefore, we should endeavor to teach rhythm, first in fast, and later in slow movements. Fast movements are frequently inhibited in dysarthric children. Consequently, we are usually compelled to progress from slow to fast. *However, we should begin with the greatest speed of which the patient is capable in order that he may sense the nature and character of rhythm.* A metronome is an excellent aid for rhythmical drill since the visual and auditory impressions derived from the pendulum are stimulating. Some patients must first learn to differentiate between slow and fast by listening to, looking at, and feeling the tapping of the therapist's fingers, a metronome, etc.

Experience has shown that exercises are often very tiresome for dysarthric patients. Hence, we must restrict every single training period to a very short span but must repeat it over and over again during the day. Each and every group of voluntary muscles should be gradually included in rhythmic drill starting first with those muscles which have been less affected and progressing to the more seriously affected muscles. Our chief interest centers about the jaw, the lips, the tongue, in fact all the muscles that constitute the speech mechanism. Shaking the jaw in advanced stages of training is, in itself, a rhythmical exercise. Similarly, the lowering and raising movements of the jaw should be rhythmical in character. The idea of rhythm must be greatly extended far beyond its normal conception in the training of dysarthric children. This is obvious, if we keep in mind the fact that they have never experienced the fundamental rhythms that are natural to normal individuals. For example, rhythm must be applied to the raising and lowering of the lower lip and to the sideward moving of the corners of the mouth, to the protruding of the lips permitting varying degrees of openness. The tongue should be given rhythmical practice in protruding and retracting, raising and lowering the tip, movement to the side, touching the corners of the mouth followed by a rhythmical drill involving the back of the tongue. Naturally, all of these movements which enter into the speech act should, in more advanced stages of training, be employed rhythmically during sound and syllable formation.

Efforts to improve the functions of the muscles of the mouth and speech organs are often accompanied by a marked decrease of salivation and drooling which frequently is exclusively due to lack of control of the closure of the mouth and a deficiency in swallowing movements. The tendency for these objectionable features to disappear is a direct result of securing a greater degree of control over the muscles involved. (See: page 121). Needless to say that listening to rhymes, music and speaking, respectively singing in rhythm, saying sounds or words to the rhythm of ball-playing are a valuable help in developing rhythmical feeling and rhythmical motions.

Palmer and *Zerbe** recommend the following observations made by *Carlson*† to help the control of athetoid movements by certain sound stimuli. After the tremor has been increased by sound stimuli, "a sudden cessation of the stimuli (rhythmic, arhythmic, musical, amusical) produced remissions of the tremor for considerable lengths of time."

The application of some methods, techniques and expedients for speech correction constitute the subject matter of the following chapter.

**Palmer, M. F.* and *Zerbe, L. E.*: "Control of Athetotic Tremors by Sound Stimuli." J. Speech Diseases, 1945, 10, pp. 303–319.

†*Carlson, E. R.*: "Infantile Cerebral Palsy; Its Treatment by Selective Inhibition of Sensory Stimuli." Amer. Intern. Med., 1937, 11, pp. 324–334. "Neurological Aspects and Treatment of Birth Injuries." New York State J. Med., 1934, 34, pp. 1–6. "Understanding and Guiding the Spastic," Am. J. Nurs. 39, pp. 356–366.

Tenth Chapter

MUSCLE TRAINING CONNECTED WITH SPEECH TRAINING

We shall now consider different techniques and procedures previously discussed which may be successfully used in improving the functions of breathing, voice production and articulation.

Mention has been made of the pathological noises produced during inhalation. They were attributed to a narrow glottis or to retraction of the back of the tongue toward the pharyngeal wall. If a narrow glottis is due to over-contraction of the closing muscles, jaw-shaking exercises are sometimes effective in such cases. It also has a favorable reaction on the contracted tongue. In other words, the noises subside or disappear altogether during the jaw-shaking exercises. If the patient does not respond to this treatment, pressure may be applied to the Adam's apple. The necessity for this should, however, be determined by the physician.

We have previously discussed the treatment of disturbed respiration and may now consider the problem of voice impairment. Here we should recall that the apparatus of the human voice is of the nature of a wind as well as a string instrument. The larynx is a kind of trumpet, the vibrating parts of which (the vocal cords) can be stretched to a greater or lesser degree. It is therefore possible that, in individual cases, training in respiration as well as training of the vocal cords may be required. Deep inhaling may be successful but only when restricted within certain limits. Over-exertion of the muscles participating in inhaling is sometimes the cause for the stiffening of other muscles and should, therefore, be avoided but a moderately deep inhalation may be useful. The air thus taken into the lungs should be emitted thriftily. The degree of loudness desired should determine the amount of breath to be used in voice production. Soft tones require less breath than loud ones. Superfluous breath adds nothing to the volume of the tone but simply accompanies it as a disturbing noise (breathy voice). In fact, breathy voice tends to diminish the loudness since the accompanying noise interferes with the tone, destroying in part the vibrations of the air which characterize tone production. Economical expiration of breath with the aid of tactile control should therefore be taught.

In singing, as well as in speaking, pitch depends chiefly upon the extent to which the vocal cords are stretched: in other words, upon the degree of tautness since the higher tones are produced with greater elongation of the vocal cords than are the lower ones.* The differences between pitches used are generally slighter in speech than in singing. This implies not only that the number of tones used in speech are fewer but also that more often, the intervals are less than a tone or a half tone, the smallest usual intervals in music. The aspects of the individual cases must determine whether greater attention should be given to increased or to decreased stretching of the vocal cords. Some patients cannot produce tone steps of more than one tone interval, while others frequently produce excessively high tones. It should be noted, however, that other patients suffering from dysarthria employ pitches greatly out of proportion which means that they jump from one pitch to another several tones higher or lower. Unfortunately, both faults may be found in one and the same individual. Here also, the therapeutic procedure will be determined by the differential diagnosis. To lessen the tension of the vocal cords, we may apply jaw-shaking exercises which will help to bring the muscles of the mouth and throat into a more natural state. During the vacillating movements of the jaw-shaking exercises, the patient should be directed to produce a vowel sound for the duration of an exhalation period. Then, after again inhaling, another vowel should be emitted. This procedure should be repeated utilizing all the vowel and diphthong sounds following

*According to the majority of writers.

which the patient should be taught to produce a series of vowel sounds such as E-A-AH-AW-O-OO with one exhalation. Immediately after the drill in voice production with accompanying jaw-shaking, the patient should be directed to repeat the same vowel or series of vowel sounds without the shaking exercises and to try to maintain relaxation of the muscles involved. The next step should be the speaking of single syllables simultaneously with the jaw-shaking exercises to be immediately followed by speaking the same syllables without the accompanying jaw-shaking. Then later on, the patient should repeat the exercises in blended syllables. Following this, we progress to monosyllabic words, then to longer words and finally to short phrases, then longer ones with accompanying jaw shaking. The latter may be stopped or started as the therapist deems necessary in the course of training.

The training of respiration is helpful in the strengthening of the vocal cords and in establishing larger intervals and increasing the number of tones. Frequently drill of diaphragmatic breathing only is recommended. Another recommendation is the use of the pushing exercises which the author introduced first for weakness of the soft palate (See page: 146). *Perlstein* and *Shere* have experienced good results with them, as well as with "chewing" and using bottle corks.* Care should be exercised in drilling the patient in "swelling tones" which play an important part in speech. Singing exercises consisting of scales, increased intervals, swelling tones, simple and gradually more complicated melodies, have a good influence on speech melody. Only vowels should be used, at least at the beginning. Some singing teachers recommend the use of the nasal sounds M or N in the voice education of normal persons. Experience has proved that while higher tones can be produced more easily with nasal sounds than with vowels, this procedure is not advisable since habitual weakness of the soft palate may result.

The chewing technique is an excellent means of freeing the voice from all kinds of muscle constriction and if the dysarthric patient suffers from such symptoms and can learn to "chew his voice," the effect should be immediate.

It is necessary to teach the patient to maintain a tone for as long a period as possible. This ability depends on slow and economic exhalation providing athetoid or choreatic movements in the mouth or face do not interrupt the stream of air.

Continued muscle training is a most effective means for the improvement of articulation and the moulding of the flow of air which results in

---

**Perlstein, M.A.* and *Shere, M.*: "Speech Therapy in Children with Cerebral Palsy." Am. J. of Diseases of Children, 72, Oct. 1946, p. 389.

fluent speech. When a patient is incapable of producing particular sounds or produces them incorrectly, he must be taught the correct formation of the phoneme by special mechanical or manual means. In many cases, the patient may imitate and practice the correct formation of the mouth by himself after it has been demonstrated and explained. Others are able to carry on the practice with the help of a mirror while in many difficult instances the therapist himself must shape the mouth. For this purpose, it is advisable to adopt the following position of the hands: with the two middle fingers the nose should be closed by side pressure on the alae nasi. The two index fingers are placed to the right and left, immediately above the ridge of the upper lips, the thumbs below the edge of the underlip. In this way, a complete ring has been formed around the lips which thus may be moved in all directions.

If the lower jaw is drawn downward, the mouth will be opened correctly for the Ah sound, as in "bar". At times, it may be necessary to press the tongue down but in most cases, it follows the movement of the lower jaw. For the A sound as in "have" only a moderate opening of the mouth should be formed. For this position of the mouth, the patient will frequently make the mistake of sounding A in a way that the indefinite vowel is produced. In this event, it is better to practice the I sound, as in "sister". For the I sound it is necessary that the corners of the mouth be drawn apart and a tongue depressor used to exercise a slight pressure on the tongue toward the roof of the mouth. In this way, the tongue is lifted upward. From the I sound one can now go to the A sound, as in "have" if the pressure is reduced and the lower jaw is drawn slightly downward. At the same time, the pull at the corners of the mouth should be relaxed.

From the Ah sound, heard in "bar", we may derive an O sound by rounding the lips since the narrow opening of the lips dulls the Ah sound and causes it to flow imperceptibly into a well-sounding O. Of all vowels, the OO, as in "too" requires the smallest opening of the mouth. A slight pressure against the floor of the mouth at the angle between the throat and the jaw produces the correct position of the tongue. By considerably narrowing the opening of the mouth, OO may be derived directly from the Ah, as in "bar" in the same way as the O sound. Diphthongs result from pronouncing the component vowels one after another in a single vocalized breath. OU, as in "house", is therefore an Ah sound as in "car" flowing into an OO sound. The IE as in "fine", is obtained with greater difficulty. Here we start from the Ah as in "car", and gradually allow the pronunciation of an I.

The best method for teaching the consonants is to proceed according to the regions of articulation.† The first region of articulation can be surveyed completely by the eye and can, therefore, be observed much more easily than the second. In the third region of articulation the eye becomes nearly useless as a means of observation.

If a patient is shown the position of the mouth in pronouncing F, he will be able to repeat the sound quite easily if he blows on his hand. A hand placed under the chin will detect no vibration with a voiceless F, but with the V, which otherwise resembles F vibrations are readily observed. A lighted candle may be utilized to demonstrate the flow of air in the formation of F. S is produced by having the patient pronounce F and while doing so the therapist and later on the patient himself moves the lips away from the teeth. (See: Chapter XI.) If the patient now adds voice to this newly learned sound, the soft Z sound is produced. From a voiceless S, the SH can be easily derived by slightly pulling the tip of the tongue backward and protruding the lips. The breath with the SH should then be compared with that of the S; the latter is thin and sharp, the former is round and full. The TH sounds are easily taught provided the patient can protrude his tongue, since the air leaving the mouth in a

†1st zone: Vowels, B, P, F, V, W, Wh, M. 2nd zone: T, D, Th (voiced and voiceless), Z, Zh, Sh, soft G, Ch, J, L, R, N. 3rd zone: G, K, Ng. The clinical picture of some individual cases might deviate from this.

continuous flow accomplishes the sound formation. If the tongue cannot be protruded but touches the upper incisors, then a modified TH will be produced. The voiced and the voiceless TH should be taught by using the patient's hand for checking the presence or absence respectively of vibrations on the therapist's throat.

The semi-vowel Y, as in "you" can be produced by blending I in "sister" with another vowel, as I-A, I-O, Y-U. When pronounced quickly the result is "ya, yo, yu."

The *plosive sounds* are P, B, D, T, K and G. The soft sounds among these are voiced. To obtain the plosive sounds of the first region of articulation the patient should be shown occlusion of the lips and be allowed to feel the escape of the breath in front of the mouth. For P a stronger occlusion and a more violent expulsion of air is necessary than for B. B contains voice which the patient should be made to feel on the larynx. If demonstration of occlusion is not successful the lips and nose may be closed with the fingers until a sufficient amount of air has been accumulated in the mouth, following which the lips should be parted. With D and T an optical demonstration of the right position in articulation is in many cases sufficient if the patient is permitted to feel the explosion simultaneously. If this expedient brings a negative result then the production of the interdental D and T is recommended. For this purpose the tongue should be placed between the incisor teeth, and then sharply moved downward with the lower jaw. Although this is a defective pronunciation it may be corrected easily later by instructing the patient first to close the teeth. The tongue then moves on its own account to the upper front teeth. During the explosion the lower jaw is pulled downward. G and K are often successfully produced by energetically pushing the tongue of the patient backward and releasing it with an explosion. One hand of the patient should be placed in front of his mouth and the other beneath the posterior part of the chin of the therapist. In this locality a short thrusting, lowering movement can be distinctly felt corresponding to the quick descent of the dorsum linguae which had been raised for the purpose of articulation. In many cases this procedure does not lead to a firm articulation between palate and dorsum linguae and a cough-like sound is produced. It should then be tried with a nasal sound of the third region of articulation: for instance, NG as in "angle." It is composed of a nasal G and an explosive G. In this, the first part acoustically resembles N, without, however, being one. From the beginning the tongue places itself in the G position. If an N (tip of the tongue touching the upper incisors) is pronounced, and the tip of the tongue is pressed to the floor of the mouth, the patient will continue to pronounce his N, while the dorsum linguae now arrives at the palate to form the occlusion. As a matter of fact, the nasal G is already before us. The nose needs only to be closed firmly and at the same time the tip of the tongue liberated, whereupon an explosive G is pronounced. Then the G so made can gradually be isolated and the patient made to conceive it as a separate sound. *Do not repeat the experiment on the first day.* The patient may begin to collaborate moving the tongue defectively. Repeat once or twice a day following the first experiment until sufficient impressions have been made on the patient to guide the tongue in voluntary collaboration.

In order to teach an L the tip of the tongue is brought to the palate and the voice is emitted. If a tongue tip R cannot be developed a uvular R may be produced by permitting the patient to feel the vibrations which the sound produces on the bottom of the therapist's mouth. At the same time slight thrusts should repeatedly be given against the dorsum linguae with the patient's index finger, from front to back while the sound is being produced. The tip of the tongue is lying on the floor of the mouth. The best position for this procedure is to have the back of the patient's head rest against the left shoulder of the therapist.

The description of this expedient for the production of correct sounds does not mean that the therapist should proceed in the order in which the sounds are described. There is a great latitude for the application of suggested techniques depending upon the clinical picture in each individual case. If the child is capable of emitting several sounds it is a question as to whether such sounds should first be corrected or whether effort should be made to establish the production of additional sounds. A general rule cannot be given. It is not wise for the therapist to restrict himself to the sounds of a definite zone of articulation, though in normal children sounds of the first and second zone of articulation in general appear earlier than those of the third, which fact seems to indicate that lip sounds and some tongue-tip sounds normally are easier to form than the sounds produced with the back of the tongue. In cerebral palsy the difficulties are markedly increased. Again, it depends upon the differential diagnosis whether it is preferable to begin with exercises of the more injured zone or with parts less affected. Every procedure is to be determined by the impression the therapist receives from the clinical picture.

There is another problem which cannot be generalized: should we begin with single sounds or with syllables? If possible we should begin with syllables or even simple words according to the normal development of speech. This order is now frequently followed with deaf children, since sounds formerly taught them singly, when later combined with other sounds were frequently characterized by unnatural modulations of the voice. On the other hand, dysarthric children are often incapable of speaking syllables, even in later stages of speech development, because of an abrupt stoppage of voice and articulation. However, if it is possible the best way is to begin with blended sounds.

If we are forced to progress from sound to syllable we often face a peculiar circumstance. Children have less difficulty in joining a foregoing vowel with a newly acquired consonant than in joining a newly learned consonant with a following vowel. For instance, they say AG more easily than GA. This difficulty may be eliminated by *Liebmann's** method. His technique is based on the observation that a vowel following a consonant is frequently slightly aspirated, which means that an inaudible H is interpolated between the consonant and the vowel. We therefore let the patient combine a consonant with vowels by interpolating an H sound; for example, B ha, B he, B hi, B ho, etc. If the patient succeeds in producing this combination quickly enough the result is practically "ba, be, bi, bo."

Of course, the aim of the therapist is to improve speech as a whole. Therefore, words and phrases must be practiced. For systematic drills the

*Vorlesungen ueber Sprachstoerungen. Coblentz, Berlin. 1925.

therapist is referred to *S. Stinchfield-Hawk** and *B. Rutherford.*†

At this point it is well to describe observations made on a patient, a boy 16 years old, a pupil in Central Institute for the Deaf, St. Louis. At the beginning some experimental phonetic methods not only revealed deficiency of the lips and tongue, but also of the soft palate. He was treated with exercises for strengthening the lips utilizing the corks previously mentioned together with exercises for the tip of the tongue consisting of rhythmic compression of a rubber ball. The boy could not hold between the lips four corks of the series, but in two months' time he was able to hold each and every one of them. In addition he developed the capacity to compress the rubber ball, an action of which he was totally incapable at the beginning. A great amount of air escaped through the nose of this patient when he spoke syllables with voiced consonants of the first and second zones of articulation. *When the muscles of the lips and tongue were strengthened by exercises, the soft palate, which had not been previously treated, effected a physiological closure between the mouth and the nose* so that it was impossible for air to pass through the nose. This surprising fact was, on the one hand, a new test for the unfavorable influence exerted

---

**l.c.*

†*Rutherford, B. R.:* "Give Them A Chance to Talk." Burges Publishing Co., 1948.

by handicapped muscles on collaborating muscles which are themselves not affected organically. On the other hand, the result described above is encouraging and evidence of the necessity to begin exercises with single muscles in order to prevent a constant hindrance of associated muscles hampered only by their defective companions. Concurrently the case indicates that a rigid therapeutic program might be upset by unexpected results.‡

---

‡*A. Bullen* reports identical experiences on non-dysarthric, but dyslalic cases. ("Nasality: Cause and Remedy of our American Blight." Quarterly J. of Speech, 1942, 28, pp. 83–84).

Eleventh Chapter

THERAPY FOR RHINOLALIA AND SIGMATISM

Treatment of Rhinolalia

Hyperrhinolalia, as we know, may be due to a cleft in the palate or to malfunctions of the soft palate. Concerning the treatment of the apertures or clefts the reader is referred to "Speech Therapy".* Malfunctions of the soft palate may be caused by actual paresis or palsy or by functional "palsy", that is a condition in which the patient lacks the motor concept to use the soft palate. In such instances, or in slight cases of actual palsy the method of *Liebmann*† may suffice. This consists of closing the nostrils during the exercise on vowels, consonants, syllables and words containing no nasal sounds. Closure of the nostrils stops the flow of air through the nose preventing the nasalized effect which is manifest in voiced sounds when the air passes through the nose. If by closure of the nostrils the air is prevented from leaving the nose, accumulated air will hinder any vibration and forward movement in

*Published by Expression Company, Magnolia, Massachusetts.

†l. c.

this cavity. On the other hand, it is impossible for additional air to find entrance into the nose. Hence the abundance of air in the pharynx will finally result in elevation of the soft palate by means of air pressure from below. In this way the patient may learn to distinguish between nasalized and non-nasalized sounds which he produces. This expedient may be utilized to teach the patient the phsyiological significance of the soft palate.

In severe cases special gymnastics for the soft palate is indicated. For this purpose the author developed a method which has proved successful in many cases of palsy of the speech mechanism. This technique is based on the physiological law that if some muscles of the body are working vigorously they are accompanied by involuntary contraction of other muscles. The patient is directed to clench the fists and to raise them to the height of the nipples, and to push down strongly yet elastically. Here we must carefully prevent vitiating mistakes. The patient may push too stiffly so that his elbows are bent at the end of the exercise; or he may thrust his hands sideward or forward. Such faults prevent the movements from being as strong and at the same time as elastic as they should be. After having systematically trained the patient in this initial exercise he should then be directed to emit a vowel *synchronously* with the downward pushing of his arms. In this stage of training two mistakes occur frequently; the vowel may be voiced before or after the downward thrust of the arms. In either case no influence on the soft palate can be expected, but if both actions are absolutely synchronous the therapist will notice very soon the favorable influence the exercise exerts on the soft palate. If the patient says AH, thus providing an opportunity to observe the action of the soft palate, the therapist will, during the exercise, often at the first attempt, see the soft palate rise to some extent. We must avoid tiring the patient. Therefore it is well to have him exercise some ten times daily for the duration of one minute. When the exercises have proved successful the patient is directed to repeat the sound without thrusting the arms immediately after he has emitted it during thrusting.

The next step will consist of utilizing single syllables (without nasal sounds) during the pushing exercise, followed by blended syllables and short words. After using the exercise for a time it will be sufficient to make one thrust of the arms simultaneously with the first syllable, while the remaining syllables in the series may be spoken without accompanying arm movements. Gradually, the patient may progress to short phrases while the number of pushing movements required will depend upon the degree of nasality which appears in his speech. This technique can, of course, be used with patients with cerebral *spastic* paralysis only when and if they are able to push the hands down forcibly, or if they can be taught to perform the exercise. Experience has shown that the exercise employing one arm is helpful if it is impossible physically to use both arms.

In extremely severe cases, or in instances where the pushing exercises cannot be employed, special medical treatment may be used. For this purpose a palato-electro masseur is recommended. (Figures 31, 32.)

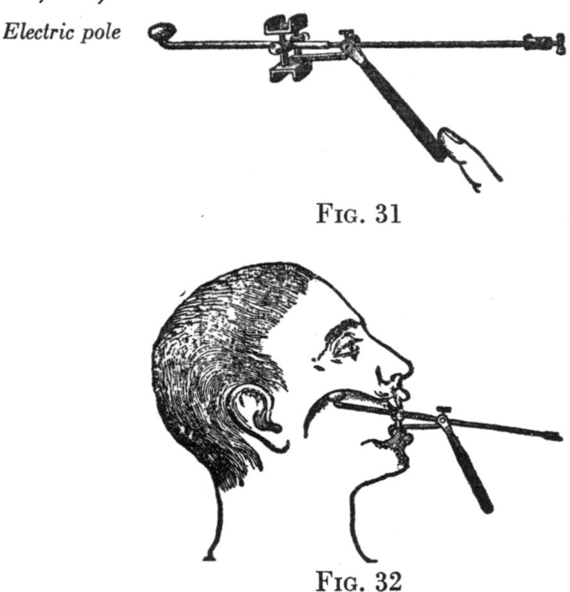

Fig. 31

Fig. 32

The second figure 32 demonstrates how the patient holds the apparatus between his teeth and how the electro pole comes in contact with the soft palate. The screw at the other end of this pole fixes one electric wire while the other pole is in contact with another part of the body, for instance, the hand. The patient or the physician may grasp the handle which is rhythmically pressed down, as shown in Fig. 31. The downward movements produce an upward pressure of the pole contacting the soft palate effecting elevation of the soft palate itself. The patient is directed *to emit a vowel the moment the soft palate is elevated.* This technique utilizing massage and electricity should be applied for ten minutes every day.

Active hyperrhinolalia requires a different treatment. Here the chewing method also seems to be the method of choice.

While the organic form of *hyporhinolalia* is a matter entirely for the rhinologist (removal of adenoids and so on) speech treatment is adequate for the *functional form.** The patient is instructed to initiate a long-drawn-out nasal sound. To assist him he is asked to feel the vibrations on the nostrils of the therapist with the fingers of one hand while endeavoring to sense the vibrations on his own nostrils with the fingers of the other hand. If the patient is capable of using only one hand he should first touch the nose of the therapist and then his own in order to feel the vibrations. If the patient succeeds in produc-

*If hyporhinolalia persists after the operation it must be considered as functional.

ing strong vibrations of the nostrils this will prove strong relaxation of the soft palate. To produce mild relaxation of those muscles the over-contraction of which is responsible for functional hyporhinolalia in voiced sounds we use "French-vowels." By this name we mean nasalized vowels which in French precede N, M, NG.** These vowels are *hyperrhinolalic* from the viewpoint of the English language. They are accompanied by vibrations of the nostrils since during their pronunciation air passes through the nose. If the patient learns to imitate them he might tend to over-relax the soft palate. Experience has shown that over-relaxation of the soft palate which initially was over-contracted, will finally result in a normal state of contraction. However, from single nasalized vowels we progress to syllables and words containing them. These exercises should be used for one to two minutes ten times a day.

Recently the writer had an opportunity to apply the *chewing method* with dysarthric children suffering from functional hyporhinolalia with satisfactory results. During chewing the soft palate rises also but not so forcibly as in speech. If the reader is informed about the chewing technique, its relation to voice and speech, and its relation to

**See: *Dantzig, B. van*: "Ueber die Funktion des Gaumensegels und des Passavant' schen Wulstes." Arch. Neerland. Pour Phonétique Experimental, 1931.

impediments of these functions, he will find another proof of the close relationship between eating and speaking in the effectiveness of the chewing treatment for hyporhinolalia.

Mixed rhinolalia is a field for combined rhinological and speech treatment. After operation on the nose treatment of the soft palate should begin.

Treatment For Sigmatism

Therapy for sigmatism depends, of course, on symptoms. If we are faced by an abnormal position of the tongue this should be treated. If it is a question of nasal or snoring sigmatism we must attempt to bring about a closing off of the oral from the nasal cavity. If the patient cannot form the S sound at all we must explain to him the correct formation of S; and by training we must facilitate and fix the correct production of the sound. *Gutzmann** corrects the *tongue position* with probes. In many cases it suffices to place a hollow key against the lower teeth having the patient blow into it. By this means a sharp S sound is obtained.

As the methods of treatment previously employed were very tiring to the patient the author has tried a method which the patient could from the beginning practice alone. A piece of

---

**Gutzmann, H.* Sprachheilkunde, 3 Auflage, Berlin, 1924.

wax (in dentistry known as "stents"), the size of the mouth, is softened in warm water and put into the patient's mouth so as to cover the lower incisors. He is directed to bite into the wax, thus making an impression of the under and upper teeth. (Fig. 33). The spaces between the teeth are filled by kneading the bits of wax jutting out

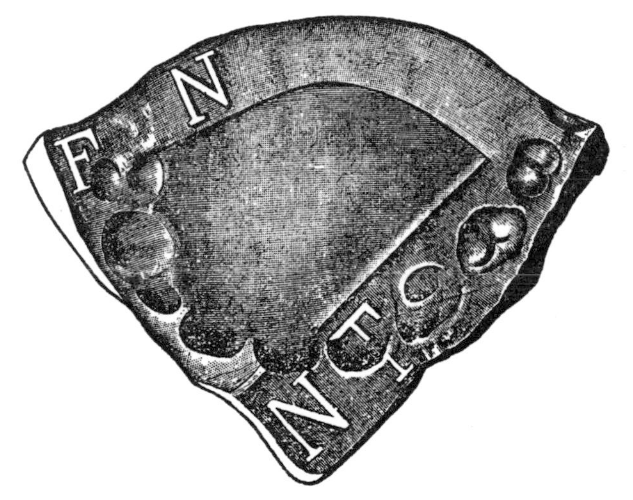

Fig. 33

through these openings. The plate is then taken out cautiously and a small rhomboid piece corresponding to the impressions of the upper middle incisors is cut out (Fig. 34). The plate is then hardened in cold water. If the patient places it in his mouth and bites into the corresponding teeth impressions the following conditions are obtained for correct pronunciation of the S sound.

1. The tongue must lie flat in the mouth as it is bridged by the plate of wax, the two jaws holding the plate together.

2. The tongue cannot overstep the row of the teeth, since the three-cornered opening in the wax plate is not large enough to permit the lifting of the front part of the tongue.

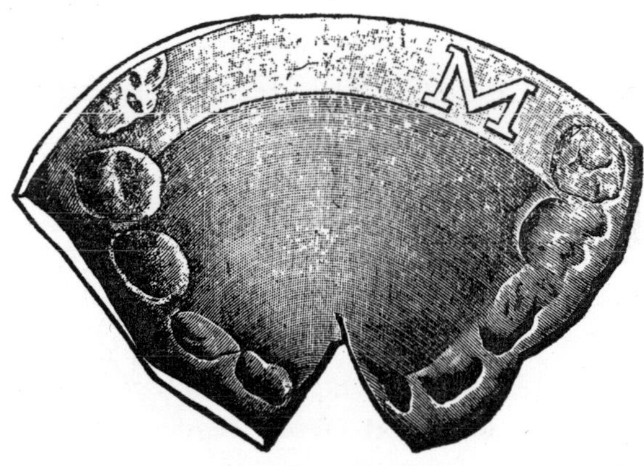

FIG. 34

3. The gaps between the teeth and the alveolar arches are closed.

4. Air can escape only through the middle of the mouth.

In many instances with this device an almost correct S resulted even upon the first use of the plate. In some cases the S sounds non-piercing (not to be confused with soft-sonant) since the air does not leave the mouth in a thin stream but escapes through the entire opening of the plate, but often this defect may be removed by demonstrating a correct S sound to the patient. In rare cases the therapist must for a time press the tongue down along the middle line with a probe until the organ assumes the correct position without the assistance of the plate. By the use of a probe the patient is aided in forming the groove for S. However, this may occur of itself as soon as the patient begins to practice without the plate. The patient should practice alone with the plate as often as possible making the periods of practice one minute in duration. The correct S sound is generally successfully made even without the use of the plate, after a few days' practice with it, provided the tongue muscles of the patient are not too greatly impaired.

The treatment of *nasal and snoring sigmatism* is essentially different from therapy of those forms resulting from false tongue position. In this type of sigmatism, action of the soft palate must be obtained and physiological direction must be given to the stream of air. A simple therapy is to have the patient blow into a small glass tube placed against the lower incisor teeth. Short practice will enable the patient to produce a satisfactory S sound if the upper lip is removed from the tube simultaneously with the act of blowing. When the new sound is definitely fixed, we can then explain to the patient that it is identical with the correct S. If there is a tendency for air to escape through the nose, this may also be corrected by exerting pressure upon the nostrils and instructing the patient to direct the entire stream of air over the grooved tongue.

A very useful technique is the transformation of F to S. The patient is directed to produce an F sound. The therapist places the index finger and thumb of each hand in both corners of the patient's mouth, pressing them between the teeth and the red of the lips, and manipulates the lips forward, upward and downward. As the air escapes from the mouth between the front teeth, the result is usually a correct S. This expedient has worked satisfactorily in all the forms of sigmatism and offers a great advantage to the therapist as it is a uniform and simple device.

During the treatment of all forms of sigmatism with any method one of two intermediate conditions may possibly develop. One condition although resembling normal S is due to an over-contraction of some muscles of the tongue, and does not lead to normal S. This resemblance to normal S may deceive the therapist. The other condition bears less resemblance to the normal S, and is caused by over-relaxation of some tongue muscles, but can be developed easily into a normal S. The following method is helpful in differentiating between the two intermediate conditions. With his thumb the therapist exerts pressure against the bottom of the mouth at the middle line close to the horizontal part of the lower jaw. If the S sound becomes sharper the therapist will recognize the presence of the useful and desirable intermediate condition. Should the S sound not become sharper overcontraction of the tongue muscles is the cause which will prevent the development of the correct S.

In nasal and snoring sigmatism, often the articulation of other continuant sounds in the second zone of articulation such as SH and CH are also similarly disturbed.

To correct a snoring SH, the therapist closes the patient's nose, instructs him to protrude his lips and directs him to puff, and at the same time exerts a slight pressure under the chin. This exercise will in time result in a correct SH sound. Often the therapist is compelled to push the tip of the tongue backward by means of a probe, or the patient may use his index finger to assist correct articulation. We should note that SH may be a defective sound even when S is correctly produced by the patient. J (f.i. in "joke") and G (f.i. in "German") contain a kind of voiced SH or ZH. The procedure is to first teach a perfect SH and only then have it voiced. CH for instance, in the word "church", is the double consonant T plus SH (voiceless).

Twelfth Chapter

COMPLICATIONS IN CEREBRAL PALSY

The reader may have expected to find a chapter on stuttering in that part of the book where the speech troubles of the dysarthric are described. However, there seems to be no reason for the assumption that the anatomic condition of the dysarthric should produce stuttering. Years of study of the stuttering problem brought the writer to the firm conviction that stuttering is entirely psychic in nature and should be included in the large classification of neuroses. Why the neurotic chooses in one instance a certain symptom, e.g. migraine and in another stuttering is still debatable. What seems to be proved is that the primary symptom of stuttering, namely, syllable repetition, is not a sign of a speech difficulty but only of a language difficulty. Children at a certain age want to talk faster than they find the words and fill that gap by repeating the last syllable or word. Such iterations show in about 80% of all children at an age of 3 to 5 years. Only about 2% use the iterations for building up the neurosis of stuttering. Rather than go into details here the reader is referred to the book,

"Twentieth Century Speech and Voice Correction."* If any real motor defect within the central nervous system were responsible for the symptoms of stuttering the stutterer would inevitably find difficulties not only at the beginning or middle but also at the end of words. *This is never the case.* (There is a certain speech trouble due to an inflammatory disease of the brain in which speech difficulties show also at the end of words. This trouble is called pallilalia.) Another fact which should be noted is that the percentage of stutterers among the dysarthrics is not greater than among non-dysarthric speakers.† If an abnormality in the central nervous system were responsible for stuttering the dysarthrics would certainly develop this speech impediment more frequently than the children without signs of cerebral palsy.

If cerebral palsy is connected with aphasia the difficult word finding which is characteristic for some forms of aphasia could lead to syllable repetition. Yet it would again be a language difficulty, exactly as in the cases mentioned above that repeat syllables.

The theory that stuttering develops because the brain lacks dominance of either side has been abandoned by most writers. A most profound

---

*Edited by *E. Froeschels.* Philosophical Library. New York. 1948.

†*Reid, L. D.* "The Frequency and Distribution of Speech Defects in Spastic Children." Master Thesis, Syracuse University, 1942.

and clear discussion of this topic can be found in *Blau's* book, "The Master Hand."* Therefore the assumption that the brain lesion in cerebral palsy may lead to lack of dominance need not be discussed in connection with stuttering. It should be mentioned that sometimes the differential diagnosis between a single spastic-dysarthric speech symptom and a single stuttering symptom may be extremely difficult and therefore can only be made by an expert.

Long experience in the treatment of stutterers with all available methods has convinced the writer that the best results can be obtained with the Chewing Method. Therefore in a case of dysarthric speech combined with stuttering the Chewing Method is the method of choice.

If feeblemindedness is joined with dysarthria the teacher of the feebleminded will probably be the first to work with the child. (About 50% to 60% of sufferers from cerebral palsy are of average intelligence. Of the remaining 50% to 40% only a few are idiots and the rest are borderline morons.) Detailed reports on thinking disorders as well as their possible improvement may be found in the book of *Strauss* and *Lehtinen*, "Psychopathology and Education of the Brain

---

**Blau, Abram:* "The Master Hand." The American Orthopsychiatric Assoc., Inc. New York. 1946.

Injured Child."* For comparison of the normal and the abnormal development see *Gesell* and *Amatruda's* book, "Developmental Diagnosis."† The teacher of the feebleminded should have some knowledge of the development of articulation. Only if and when the mental state is improved can the speech specialist be called on to help. There is some hope for these unfortunate cases. This hope is founded on the possibility that the general picture may be caused partly by the inability to speak. Speech is not only a means of utterance but also the way to acquire and organize knowledge. With the acquisition of speech the way may be opened to gradual improvement. The hard work done by the physician, the teacher, the speech therapist, the mother and/or the nurse, may be rewarded in spite of the severity of the initial clinical picture.

Epileptic seizures are a very severe, but fortunately, not frequent complication of cerebral palsy. Three forms of these seizures may occur. The unilateral form in which only one side is involved (Jackson's cramps), the form which affects both sides of the body and during which the patient is always unconscious (the duration of the seizures of both of these forms is usually a period of at least a few minutes) and the form

***A. A. Strauss. L. E. Lehtinen.* Grune and Stratten. New York. 1947.

†*A. Gesell. C. S. Armatruda.* P. B. Hoeber. New York. 1941. p. 231.

known as "petit mal" characterized by shortness of duration (a few seconds) and, as a rule, by absence of cramps. During petit mal seizure the patient may suddenly cease activity, the head may drop, and the eyes become fixed. At times his behavior may change abruptly, and he may iterate a few words, and there may be loss of stool and urine. Afterwards the patient may continue his activity without knowing of his seizure.

Emotional instability is a frequent complication in spastic cerebral palsy. Sudden outbreaks of unmotivated laughing or crying are phenomena which some writers relate to emotional centers localized in the neighborhood of the striatum pallidum. Fits of depression or bad temper are frequently characteristic of this malady. Adults with a lesion of a certain part of the frontal brain change their character. In early childhood not much will show along these lines except unusual behavior. These complications will naturally aggravate the clinical picture and impede the therapeutic attempts. Only general educative measures to calm the child and perhaps some medical prescriptions (sedatives) may be effective.

Deafness or hardness of hearing are serious complications. According to *Rutherford** 41%

**B. R. Rutherford.* "Hearing Loss in Cerebral Palsied Children." Journ. Speech Disorders. 10, 3, Sept. 1945. pp. 237–240. Also A Comparative Study of Loudness, Pitch, Rate, Rhythm and Quality of Children Handicapped by Cerebral Palsy. Ibidem 9, 3, Sept. 1944. p. 263–271.

suffer from hearing loss, mostly in the high frequency range. For more thorough discussion of this problem the reader is referred to *M. A. Goldstein's*† book, "Problems of the Deaf." Audiometry is often not reliable with children, therefore it is advisable to use the method of "direct tone introduction" which is described in "Twentieth Century Speech and Voice Correction."‡ *Urbantschitsch* constructed an accordion the bellows of which can be fitted with single whistles. These whistles comprise 6 octaves. If one puts a rubber tube on the small opening of a whistle and puts the other end of the tube into the patient's ear (via an ear olive) a very obvious reflex of the face usually results if the patient hears the particular tone which is being tested. Negative results reported in many cases tested with audiometry have been proved incorrect when the patients have been tested with direct tone introduction.** Rare cases of hardness of hearing may be central (psychogenic) in nature. The reader is referred to the article, "Psychogenic Deafness in Children."§

---

†*Max A. Goldstein.* The Laryngoscope Press. St. Louis, Mo.

‡l. c. p. 205 ff.

**It remains to be seen whether the Psycho-Galvanic Skin Test can be used in dysarthrics. See: Hardy, W. G. and Bordley, J. E. A Study in Objective Audiometry with the use of a Psychogalvanometric Response. Annals of Otology and Laryngology. Vol. 58, 3 Sept. 1949. pp. 1–9.

§*E. Froeschels.* Archives of Neurology and Psychiatry. June 1944. Vol. 51, pp. 544–549.

A tragic complication of cerebral spastic palsy is blindness. Here reference is made to *Stinchfield-Hawk's*° profound studies on the problem of blindness in children.

Persons without experience in the pathology and therapy of dysarthrics might not only be confused by the variety of clinical pictures but also pessimistic as to the possibility of improvement. A great number of signs and symptoms do not necessarily indicate the severity of a given case. Therefore, those engaged in the treatment of a dysarthric patient should not be discouraged by the complexity of the clinical picture. Many difficulties involved in the efforts at improving dysarthrics have been discussed. Nevertheless, the reader may be sure that the author would not have made the endeavor to present comprehensive descriptions of many of the symptoms and the therapeutic methods had it not been his experience that the majority of cases can be helped. Improving dysarthric speech carries a special reward with it — the whole personality may become more sociable, less depressed, more optimistic, less "nervous", as is the case with many non-dysarthrics who have been relieved from various speech and voice difficulties.

°*S. Stinchfield-Hawk.* "The Blind Child of Pre-School Age and His Speech." The Nervous Child. 9, 1. January 1951. pp. 48–56.

SOME ADDITIONAL LITERATURE

BERGER, CLYDE C. "Subjective Observations on Cerebral Palsy." Journ. of Speech Disorders. 10, Dec. 1945. pp. 297–302.

BOUMAN, H. D., SCHWARTZ, R. P. "The Degree, Extent, and the Mechanism of Muscle Spasm in Infantile Paralysis." N. Y. State Journ. of Med. 44, No. 2, Jan 15, 1944. pp. 147–151.

CARLSON, E. R. "Treatment of Infantile Cerebral Palsy." The Diplomate. XV June–July 1943. pp. 201–205.

DE HIRSCH, K. "Speech Therapy in Children with Cerebral Palsy." Folia Phoniatrica. Vol. 2, 1, 1949. p. 56. Evan, M. F. "Children with Cerebral Palsy" in Johnson, E. W. "Speech Problems of Children." New York, 1950.

HICKS, S. P. "Brain Repair." Southern Med. Journ. 41, 7. July 1948. pp. 581–586.

HOOD, P. N., SHANK, K. H., WILLIAMSON, D. B. "Environmental Factors in Relation to the Speech of Cerebral Palsied Children." Journ. of Speech and Hearing Disorders. 13, 4, Dec. 1948. pp. 325–331.

LASSEK, A. M. "The Human Pyramidal Tract." Arch. of Neurol. and Psych. 52, 6, Dec. 1944. pp. 484–494.

LITTLE, CH. "Investigations of Emotional Complications in Cerebral Palsy." The Nervous Child. 8, 2. April 1949. pp. 181–182.

MUSSAFIA, M. "Le langage du Parkinsonien." Scalpel. No. 1, Jan. 1947.

O'BRIEN, V. "Treatment of Children with Cerebral Palsy." N. Y. State Med. Journ. July 15, 1945. pp. 1548–1550.

OGINO, P. "Anatomic Explanation of Dysarthria." Psychiatry and Neurology Japanese. Vol. 39, 27.

PEACHER, W. O. "The Etiology and Differential Diagnosis of Dysarthria." Journ. of Speech Disorders. 15, 3. Sept. 1950. pp. 252–265.

SCHILLING, R. "Ein Fall von Choreatischer Dysarthrie." Monatschrift fuer Ohrenheilkunde und Laryngo-Rhinologie. Vol. 66. 1932.

SEEMANN, M. "Les Troubles de la Parole dans la Maladie de Wilson." Societé Tchechoslov. d'otol. May 15, 1937.

INDEX

INDEX OF AUTHORS